BOTTOM LINE'S

AGELESS HEALTH, AGELESS BEAUTY

FROM THE EDITORS OF BOTTOM LINE PUBLICATIONS

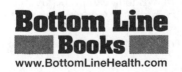

Bottom Line Books

www.BottomLineHealth.com

Contents

Preface

We are proud to bring you *Ageless Health, Ageless Beauty*. What you are holding in your hand is a collection of solutions for your everyday health problems and discomforts. Whether it's arthritis pain, fibromyalgia, headaches, sexual dysfunction, insomnia or emotional stress (and much more), our editors talk to the true innovators in women's health care to find the best answers to all your health questions.

How do we find all these top-notch medical professionals? Over the past two decades, we have built a network of literally thousands of leading physicians in both alternative and conventional medicine. They are affiliated with the premier medical institutions and the best universities throughout the world. We read the important medical journals and follow the latest research reported at medical conferences. And we regularly talk to our advisors in major teaching hospitals, private practices and government health agencies.

Ageless Health, Ageless Beauty is a result of our ongoing research and contact with these experts, and is a distillation of their latest findings and advice. We trust that you will enjoy the presentation and glean new, helpful and affordable information about the health topics that concern you and your family.

As a reader of a Bottom Line book, please be assured that you are receiving reliable and well-researched information from a trusted source. But, please use prudence in health matters. Always speak to your physician before taking vitamins, supplements or over-the-counter medication...changing your diet...or beginning an exercise program. If you experience side effects from any regimen, contact your doctor immediately.

The Editors, Bottom Line Publications
Stamford, Connecticut

Arthritis Relief

Natural Cures for Arthritis: Research Shows They Really Work!

If you have arthritis, you may have shied away from natural medicine in the past because you didn't think that it would relieve your pain.

After all, there is no rigorous scientific evidence to back up these remedies, right?

Wrong.

Now: While it's true that many nondrug approaches for pain relief have been based primarily on their thousands of years of use by Asian, Indian and other traditional cultures, there is now an impressive body of scientific evidence that makes natural medicine a smarter choice than ever before for many arthritis sufferers. (These therapies have been studied most often for osteoarthritis but may also relieve pain due to rheumatoid arthritis. Check with your doctor.)

PAIN RELIEF WITH LESS RISK

Millions of Americans depend on high-dose pain relievers that cause side effects, including gastrointestinal upset or bleeding, in up to 60% of patients.

What you may not realize is that some natural therapies, which are far less likely to cause side effects, work just as well as the powerful pain-relieving drugs that are so commonly used for arthritis.

Many Americans take glucosamine (a dietary supplement that stimulates production of key components in cartilage) to help fight arthritis. However, arthritis pain symptoms improve only slightly or moderately in some patients—even when they take glucosamine sulfate, the most widely studied form of this supplement. (Research currently indicates that adding

Steven Ehrlich, NMD, a naturopathic physician and founder of Solutions Acupuncture & Naturopathic Medicine in Phoenix. He has spent the last decade using natural medicine to treat chronic pain and illness. Dr. Ehrlich has also taught naturopathic techniques to both conventional and alternative medicine practitioners.

chondroitin, a supplement derived from shark or bovine cartilage or produced synthetically, isn't necessarily helpful for arthritis).

In my practice, I often recommend the following regimen (with or without glucosamine) to relieve arthritis pain—the typical arthritis patient might start with curcumin and fish oil (pain relief should begin within one week to a month). *Ginger can be added if more pain relief is needed…*

●**Curcumin.** A chemical compound in the spice turmeric, it helps inhibit inflammatory enzymes and reduces joint pain without the gastrointestinal side effects that often occur with aspirin and related drugs.

Scientific evidence: A study published in *The Journal of Alternative and Complementary Medicine* found that curcumin reduced arthritis pain and improved knee function about as well as *ibuprofen* (Motrin).

How to use curcumin: To obtain a concentrated dose of the active ingredient, try curcumin supplement capsules with a standardized curcuminoid complex (rather than kitchen turmeric, which would be difficult to consume in therapeutic amounts). Follow the label instructions—typically taking it three times daily during flare-ups. Between arthritis episodes, you can take half this amount to prevent inflammation.

Caution: Curcumin can inhibit the ability of blood to clot. Use this supplement only under a doctor's supervision, particularly if you're also taking a blood-thinning medication such as *warfarin* (Coumadin) or aspirin.

●**Fish oil.** The omega-3 fatty acids in fish oil supplements increase the body's production of inhibitory prostaglandins, substances that prevent inflammation.

Scientific evidence: A study published in *Arthritis & Rheumatism* discovered that some arthritis patients who took fish oil improved so much that they were able to discontinue their use of conventional painkillers.

How to use fish oil: The amount of omega-3s found in dietary sources is insufficient for pain relief. Use a fish oil supplement—doses range from about 2,000 mg to 6,000 mg daily. Start with the lower dose, then gradually increase it until you notice improvement in pain and stiffness (the rate at which the dose is increased depends on the patient). If you take more than 2,000 mg of fish oil daily, you should be monitored by a physician—this supplement has a blood-thinning effect.

●**Ginger.** This spice has compounds that inhibit the effects of cyclooxygenase, an inflammatory enzyme.

Scientific evidence: A study that looked at 261 patients with knee arthritis discovered that those who took ginger supplements had less pain—and required fewer painkillers—than those taking placebos.

How to use ginger: Ginger spice will not provide enough of the active ingredient, so use a ginger supplement. The standard dose is 250 mg taken four times daily. Talk to your doctor before trying ginger—especially if it's used with a blood-thinning drug, curcumin and/or fish oil. Ginger can increase the risk for bleeding in some patients.

OTHER THERAPIES THAT HELP

The following approaches can accelerate and increase the pain-relieving effects offered by the supplements described earlier…

●**Balance Method acupuncture.** Acupuncture can be extremely effective because it increases the flow of blood and oxygen into painful areas while accelerating the removal of inflammatory chemicals.

Scientific evidence: A study involving more than 3,500 patients with chronic hip and/or knee arthritis found that those given acupuncture (in addition to conventional care, including doctor visits and use of painkillers) had fewer symptoms and a better quality of life than those given only conventional treatments.

My advice: Consider trying Balance Method acupuncture. Rather than inserting needles above or near the painful areas (as occurs with standard acupuncture), the practitioner will use

---

*Consult a doctor before trying these supplements—especially if you have a chronic condition or take medication. To find a physician near you with experience prescribing botanical medicines, consult the American Association of Naturopathic Physicians at *naturopathic. org*

points on your arms or legs that "remotely" affect the joints. It seems to be more effective than standard acupuncture.

How acupuncture is used: Virtually all arthritis patients improve by the end of the third session—some after the first session. Most practitioners advise an initial series of 12 to 15 sessions, given once or twice a week, followed by monthly "tune-ups."

● **Meditation.** Meditation works in part by lowering levels of stress hormones. This decreases inflammation as well as the perception of pain. Patients who do meditation may still have pain, but it won't bother them as much as it did before.

Scientific evidence: In a study reported at an American College of Rheumatology meeting, arthritis patients who did meditation for 45 minutes a day, six days a week for six months had an 11% decrease in symptoms, a 46% decrease in erythrocyte sedimentation rate (a measure of inflammation) and a 33% reduction in psychological stress.

How meditation is used: Practice meditation for five to 10 minutes, once or twice a day—even during symptom-free periods.

Helpful: "Tapping meditation," which incorporates elements of acupressure as the patient taps different areas of his/her body. It has been especially helpful for arthritis patients in my practice. Most health practitioners who recommend meditation can teach you how to perform tapping meditation.

● **Yoga.** Any form of exercise is helpful for arthritis as long as it doesn't put excessive pressure on the joints. Yoga is particularly beneficial because it gently stretches and strengthens the muscles. It also increases the movement of synovial (lubricating) fluid across bone surfaces.

Scientific evidence: Researchers recently found that patients with knee osteoarthritis who took a weekly yoga class had improvements in pain and mobility after just eight weeks.

How yoga is used: The yoga that's practiced in many health clubs and yoga studios may be too aggressive for patients who have arthritis. Start with a beginner's class, prefera-

bly one that's taught by an instructor who specializes in therapeutic yoga, which is designed to treat specific medical conditions. To find a yoga instructor who specializes in therapeutic yoga, consult the International Association of Yoga Therapists at *www.iayt.org*.

Prolotherapy Sugar Injections Relieve Knee Arthritis Pain

David Rabago, MD, associate professor, department of family medicine and community health, University of Wisconsin School of Medicine and Public Health, Madison.

If you find yourself carefully maneuvering up and down stairs and in and out of chairs because your knees are so painful and stiff, your doctor may have diagnosed osteoarthritis, the "wear and tear" type of arthritis. Exercise helps alleviate the stiffness but can be too uncomfortable for some sufferers…and painkilling drugs provide only temporary relief while carrying a risk for potentially serious side effects.

The good news: There's promising new evidence that an alternative treatment requiring just a few visits to a doctor's office can ease symptoms for a year or more. It makes use of a substance you normally wouldn't consider to be therapeutic—sugar!

The treatment involves injecting a solution into and around painful joints. Called prolotherapy, the technique has been around for at least 75 years. However, it isn't broadly accepted because there haven't been many high-quality studies demonstrating its effectiveness and clarifying which type of solution works best. *With the recent publication of a study from the University of Wisconsin School of Medicine, that may be about to change…*

SWEET SOLUTION

The study included 90 adults with osteoarthritis of the knee and moderate-to-severe pain that had lasted for at least three months and had not responded well to other treatments. At the start of the study, all participants completed questionnaires that assessed, using a 100-point scale, the severity of their arthritis in terms of pain, stiffness and loss of function.

Next, participants were randomly assigned to one of three groups. One group was instructed in knee exercises and encouraged to practice them at home, gradually working their way up over the course of 20 weeks until they were doing the exercises three times during the day, five days per week.

Participants in groups two and three received prolotherapy sessions at weeks one, five and nine…and at weeks 13 and 17 if the participant and his/her physician thought the additional treatment would be helpful. Group two received injections of a saline (salt) solution… group three received injections of a dextrose (sugar) solution. Each session included up to 15 injections. Because this was a "blinded" experiment, neither the participants nor the doctor giving the injections knew which type of solution was being used on any given patient.

At several points during the treatment and a year after the start of the study, participants again filled out the symptom questionnaires to score their pain, stiffness and function.

Results: The dextrose prolotherapy group had the best improvement by a significant margin. Nine weeks into the study, after the third round of prolotherapy, the dextrose group's symptom score had improved by 13.9 points, on average. In comparison, the saline prolotherapy group had improved by 6.8 points… and the exercise group improved by an average of just 2.5 points.

Even more encouraging was the fact that the relief seemed to be long-lasting. Though the final injections were given at week nine, 13 or 17 (depending on the patient), at week 52 the dextrose prolotherapy group still reported an average improvement of 15.3 points compared with their pretreatment symptom scores. This degree of improvement on the 100-point scale has been determined to be "clinically robust" in prior studies, the researchers said. In comparison, the saline prolotherapy group wound

up with an average improvement of just 7.6 points, while the exercise group ended up with an 8.2-point improvement.

How it works: No one knows exactly how prolotherapy helps or why the sugar solution would work better than the salt solution. The basic theory, though, is that the injections provoke minor, temporary inflammation, causing the body to send more blood and nutrients to the area and thus promoting a healing response.

NOT-ENTIRELY-PAINLESS PAIN TREATMENT

Although the anesthetic lidocaine was used to minimize the discomfort of the injections, participants reported short-term mild-to-moderate pain as the shots were given. No other adverse side effects were noted. The temporary discomfort seemed to be worth it, though— among participants who received dextrose prolotherapy, 91% said that they would recommend the treatment to other people with knee arthritis.

The procedure also can hurt the wallet—because most insurance providers do not cover prolotherapy, considering it to be experimental. If paying out-of-pocket, you can expect dextrose prolotherapy to cost from about $150 to $500 per session, depending on the provider and location. Still, you may consider that money well-spent if it brings significant relief from pain and allows you to once again participate in everyday activities and favorite pastimes.

Prolotherapy should be administered by a physician (an MD, ND or DO) trained in the procedure. Ask your primary care doctor for a referral, or check the provider locator of the American Association of Orthopaedic Medicine, then call the doctor you are considering to find out whether he uses dextrose solution. You may be advised to temporarily reduce or discontinue anti-inflammatory drugs (aspirin, ibuprofen, naproxen) while undergoing prolotherapy—but acetaminophen is OK if it's otherwise safe for you. If you take blood thinners or other drugs, tell the doctor because extra precautions may be warranted.

Slow Rheumatoid Arthritis with Early Detection

Beth L. Jonas, MD, associate professor of medicine and director of the Rheumatology Fellowship Program at the University of North Carolina Thurston Arthritis Research Center in Chapel Hill.

A n elderly woman has fingers so gnarled and painful that she can scarcely hold a fork. The cause is rheumatoid arthritis (RA). When she told her doctor that her middle-aged daughter was starting to show signs of the disease, he urged, "Tell your daughter to see a doctor right away."

Why the rush? Because now there are ways to limit the disease's progression, most notably with *disease-modifying antirheumatic drugs* (DMARDs). But these work best when treatment begins within six to 12 weeks of the onset of symptoms.

Unfortunately, many RA sufferers postpone seeking medical care...and once they do, doctors may not accurately diagnose the disease or may fail to refer patients to rheumatologists, the specialists best equipped to treat RA. In a recent study in *Arthritis & Rheumatism*, 69% of RA patients did not see a rheumatologist within those crucial first 12 weeks—and the delay contributed to a 30% faster rate of joint destruction and an 87% lower likelihood of remission, compared with patients who saw a specialist promptly.

"Permanent joint damage can occur at a very early stage of the disease. Medication can slow and sometimes prevent joint destruction—but once damage is done, we can't reverse it," Beth L. Jonas, MD, director of the Rheumatology Fellowship Program at the University of North Carolina Thurston Arthritis Research Center, said.

New concern: Some research links the high levels of inflammation associated with RA to cardiovascular disease, Dr. Jonas said.

What about people who have already missed that window of opportunity for early treatment? Avoiding further delay is vital because the new medications still can help somewhat...whereas RA sufferers left untreated face a significantly increased risk of becoming disabled.

SPOTTING THE SIGNS

With RA, the immune system attacks the synovial membranes that line the joints. This lining becomes inflamed and thickened...fluid builds up...ligaments and tendons weaken and stretch out...cartilage is destroyed... and bone is damaged. Over time, patients develop crippling chronic pain and joint deformity.

Women are two to three times more likely than men to get RA. The disease can arise at any time but usually appears in midlife. While genetics may play some role, most RA patients have no close relatives with the disease—so we all should be on the lookout for RA. *See your doctor without delay if you experience any of the following...*

• **Pain,** tenderness and/or stiffness in any of the small joints—fingers, wrists, toes, ankles—usually occurring symmetrically on both sides of the body. (As RA progresses, the neck, shoulders, elbows, hips and/or knees also may be affected.)

• **Morning stiffness** that lasts for more than 30 minutes.

• **Redness,** swelling and/or sensations of heat at the joints.

• **Numbness,** tingling or burning sensations in the hands or feet.

Confirming an RA diagnosis can be tricky because the symptoms mimic those of lupus, Lyme disease and other forms of arthritis. Diagnosis is based on a physical exam...blood tests for antibodies (including rheumatoid factor and anti-cyclic citrullinated peptide) plus various markers of inflammation...and imaging tests (ultrasound, MRI, X-ray).

So if your doctor suspects RA, ask to be referred to a rheumatologist or get a referral through the American College of Rheumatology (visit *www.rheumatology.org* and click on "Find a Rheumatologist").

White Willow Bark Fights Osteoarthritis

It contains salicin, a pain reliever similar to the analgesic in aspirin. White willow bark takes longer to start working than aspirin, but its effects generally last longer.

Usual dose: A standardized willow bark extract containing 100 milligrams of salicin (in capsule or tablet form) two or three times a day.

Caution: Avoid willow bark if you have ulcers or stomach problems or are allergic to aspirin.

Laurie Steelsmith, ND, naturopathic physician and acupuncturist based in Honolulu and author of *Natural Choices for Women's Health. DrSteelsmith.com*

Better Osteoarthritis Treatment

Brian Feagan, MD, director, clinical trials, Robarts Research Institute, University of Western Ontario, London, Ontario.

According to a recent finding, when 178 patients with moderate-to-severe osteoarthritis of the knee were treated with physical therapy and medical therapy, including anti-inflammatory drugs…or arthroscopic surgery (in which lens-equipped instruments are used to repair knee joint problems), the surgery provided no additional benefit (related to joint pain, stiffness and function) over medical therapy in the next two years.

If you have knee osteoarthritis: Ask your doctor whether physical therapy, along with medications (such as nonsteroidal anti-inflammatory drugs), if necessary, would benefit you.

ARTHRITIS SUPPLEMENTS DO HELP

Many patients have asked me about the well-publicized Glucosamine/Chondroitin Arthritis Intervention Trial. This six-month, multicenter clinical trial tested glucosamine and chondroitin as a treatment for knee osteoarthritis. In the study, 1,583 participants (average age 59) with knee osteoarthritis pain were randomly assigned to one of five treatment groups for 24 weeks: Glucosamine alone (1,500 mg per day)…chondroitin alone (1,200 mg)…glucosamine and chondroitin (1,500 mg and 1,200 mg, respectively)…200 mg of the prescription anti-inflammatory drug *celecoxib* (Celebrex)… or a placebo.

Researchers concluded that "glucosamine and chondroitin sulfate alone or in combination did not reduce pain effectively in the overall group of patients with osteoarthritis of the knee." As a result, many media outlets reported that glucosamine and chondroitin were ineffective for the treatment of osteoarthritis. While the combination wasn't effective for mild sufferers in the study, it was more effective than Celebrex for participants with moderate to severe osteoarthritis pain of the knees. Yet most of the mainstream media did not report this finding. Interestingly, for the group of patients with moderate to severe pain, Celebrex was only mildly more effective than the placebo.

My view: If you are being helped by these supplements, keep taking them. It's also worthwhile to try them before taking Celebrex or a similar drug, since glucosamine and chondroitin have a much lower risk of side effects, such as digestive upset. Even if you have only mild pain, these supplements can help prevent cartilage breakdown so that the problem does not worsen. For high-quality formulas, use brands sold at health-food stores.

Caution: Glucosamine and chondroitin may increase insulin resistance, so people with diabetes should monitor blood sugar levels carefully. The combination supplement should not be used by people with shellfish allergies.

Breakthrough Research On Beating Arthritis Pain Naturally

Peter Bales, MD, a board-certified orthopedic surgeon and author of *Osteoarthritis: Preventing and Healing Without Drugs.*

Osteoarthritis has long been considered a "wear-and-tear" disease associated with age-related changes that occur within cartilage and bone.

Now: A growing body of evidence shows that osteoarthritis may have a metabolic basis. Poor diet results in inflammatory changes and damage in cartilage cells, which in turn lead to cartilage breakdown and the development of osteoarthritis.

A recent increase in osteoarthritis cases corresponds to similar increases in diabetes and obesity, other conditions that can be fueled by poor nutrition. Dietary approaches can help prevent—or manage—all three of these conditions.

Key scientific evidence: A number of large studies, including many conducted in Europe as well as the US, suggest that a diet emphasizing plant foods and fish can support cartilage growth and impede its breakdown. People who combine an improved diet with certain supplements can reduce osteoarthritis symptoms—and possibly stop progression of the disease.

A SMARTER DIET

By choosing your foods carefully, you can significantly improve the pain and stiffness caused by osteoarthritis. *How to get started...*

•**Avoid acidic foods.** The typical American diet, with its processed foods, red meat and harmful trans-fatty acids, increases acidity in the body. A high-acid environment within the joints increases free radicals, corrosive molecules that both accelerate cartilage damage and inhibit the activity of cartilage-producing cells known as chondrocytes.

•**A Mediterranean diet,** which includes generous amounts of fruits, vegetables, whole grains, olive oil and fish, is more alkaline. (The body requires a balance of acidity and alkalinity, as measured on the pH scale.) A predominantly alkaline body chemistry inhibits free radicals and reduces inflammation.

What to do: Eat a Mediterranean-style diet, including six servings daily of vegetables... three servings of fruit...and two tablespoons of olive oil. (The acids in fruits and vegetables included in this diet are easily neutralized in the body.) Other sources of healthful fats include olives, nuts (such as walnuts), canola oil and flaxseed oil or ground flaxseed.

Important: It can take 12 weeks or more to flush out acidic toxins and reduce arthritis symptoms after switching to an alkaline diet.

•**Limit your intake of sugary and processed foods.** Most Americans consume a lot of refined carbohydrates as well as sugar-sweetened foods and soft drinks—all of which damage joints in several ways. For example, sugar causes an increase in advanced glycation endproducts (AGEs), protein molecules that bind to collagen (the connective tissue of cartilage and other tissues) and make it stiff and brittle. AGEs also appear to stimulate the production of cartilage-degrading enzymes.

What to do: Avoid processed foods, such as white flour (including cakes, cookies and crackers), white pasta and white rice, as well as soft drinks and fast food. Studies have shown that people who mainly eat foods in their whole, natural forms tend to have lower levels of AGEs and healthier cartilage.

Important: Small amounts of sugar—used to sweeten coffee or cereal, for example—will not significantly increase AGE levels.

•**Get more vitamin C.** More than 10 years ago, the Framingham study found that people who took large doses of vitamin C had a three-fold reduction in the risk for osteoarthritis progression.

Vitamin C is an alkalinizing agent due to its anti-inflammatory and antioxidant properties. It blocks the inflammatory effects of free radicals. Vitamin C also decreases the formation of AGEs and reduces the chemical changes that cause cartilage breakdown.

What to do: Take a vitamin C supplement (1,000 mg daily for the prevention of osteoarthritis...2,000 mg daily if you have osteoarthritis).* Also increase your intake of vitamin C–rich foods, such as sweet red peppers, strawberries and broccoli.

• **Drink green tea.** Green tea alone won't relieve osteoarthritis pain, but people who drink green tea and switch to a healthier diet may notice an additional improvement in symptoms. That's because green tea is among the most potent sources of antioxidants, including catechins, substances that inhibit the activity of cartilage-degrading enzymes.

For osteoarthritis, drink one to two cups of green tea daily. (Check with your doctor first if you take any prescription drugs.)

• **Eat fish.** Eat five to six three-ounce servings of omega-3–rich fish (such as salmon, sardines and mackerel) weekly. Omega-3s in such fish help maintain the health of joint cartilage and help curb inflammation. If you would prefer to take a fish oil supplement rather than eat fish, see the recommended dosage on page 2.

*Check with your doctor before taking any dietary supplements.

How People With Arthritis Can Avoid Joint Replacement

Kimberly Beauchamp, ND, licensed naturopathic doctor and health and nutrition writer. *KimberlyBeauchamp.com*

Arthritis is easily the most common cause of physical disability in America. The Centers for Disease Control and Prevention says that 52.5 million Americans have doctor-diagnosed arthritis (including both osteoarthritis, or OA, and rheumatoid arthritis, or RA) and predicts that that number will soar to 67 million in the next 20 years. That's a lot of stiff, painful knees, hands, shoulders and feet!

While some folks joke that they're headed straight for joint replacement, the truth is that arthritis responds well to many natural therapies, including dietary supplements. We contacted Kimberly Beauchamp, ND, a licensed naturopathic physician and health and nutrition writer who treats many arthritis patients.

PAIN SOOTHERS FOR ARTHRITIS PATIENTS

Dr. Beauchamp shared some supplements and natural therapies that many arthritis patients find helpful...

• **Zyflamend.** This proprietary blend of supplements* contains 10 anti-inflammatory plant extracts that can be helpful for many people with both OA and RA. Dr. Beauchamp has patients take one capsule twice daily with meals. (Available online at *www.newchapter.com* and at many health-food stores.)

• **Red Seaweed Extract.** Red seaweed extract (Lithothamnion calcareum) can help people with OA. One study reported in *Nutrition Journal* and funded by Marigot, the company that makes Aquamin (a patented red seaweed extract), found that taking the extract for one month was associated with a 20% reduction in arthritis pain. Patients also reported less stiffness and better range of motion and were able to walk further than those taking a placebo. A typical dose would be 2,400 mg of seaweed extract in capsule form each day, Dr. Beauchamp said. (Note: Seaweed contains iodine in amounts that may be dangerous to thyroid patients.)

• **Vitamin D.** New research indicates that vitamin D may play a key role in slowing the development and progression of both OA and RA. If you have either, it's a good idea to get your blood level of vitamin D checked, said Dr. Beauchamp. If you are deficient, she suggests taking at least 1,000 IU of vitamin D-3 (cholecalciferol) each day.

• **Peat/Peloid Packs** (also called balneotherapy). Commonly used in Europe, this is a form of thermal mud therapy that holds heat particularly well. Peat (or peloid packs that are

*Check with your doctor before using the herb and supplement mentioned in this article for medicinal purposes. The natural compounds found in herbs and spices may interact with some prescription drugs. Pregnant and nursing women should avoid using spices medicinally.

sheets of peat mud on fabric) is applied to the aching area for about 20 minutes. The treatment can be done at home, but Dr. Beauchamp said it is far better to work with a physical therapist or doctor who is knowledgeable in the technique, as the packs are cumbersome and must be carefully applied to protect the skin from burning. Peat therapy treatments are typically administered over the course of several visits, declining in frequency as the patient's pain begins to ease—the results are long-lasting and you can resume treatment if and when the pain returns.

Oregano for Arthritis

James A. Duke, PhD, an economic botanist retired from the USDA, where he developed a database on the health benefits of various plants (*www.ars-grin.gov/ duke*). He is the author of numerous books including, most recently, *The Green Pharmacy Guide to Healing Foods: Proven Natural Remedies to Treat and Prevent More Than 80 Common Health Concerns.*

O regano helps alleviate osteoarthritis and other inflammatory conditions, such as rheumatoid arthritis. You might be surprised to learn that this favorite spice of Italian cooking contains natural compounds that have many of the same effects as the powerful anti-inflammatory COX-2 inhibitor drug *celecoxib* (Celebrex).

In addition, oregano contains dozens of other anti-inflammatory compounds that act as muscle relaxants and pain relievers. Unlike celecoxib, which may increase heart attack risk in some people, oregano actually protects the heart by helping to prevent blood clots and irregular heart rhythms.

Best uses: Use oregano liberally on salads or on pizzas. Oregano also can be mixed with peppermint and/or spearmint for a hot or iced mixed-herb tea. If you prefer to take an anti-inflammatory supplement, oregano is one of the half dozen spices in a product called Zyflamend (its ingredients also include rosemary and turmeric). The herbs in Zyflamend act synergistically to provide a more powerful effect than each would when used individually. Zyflamend can be purchased in health-food stores and online. Follow label instructions.

Natural Rx for Arthritis

H ere's a soothing tea for arthritis pain… Bring one-half cup of water to a boil. Add fresh ginger, cut into thin slices—you can use as much as you like—and let simmer for five minutes. Remove and discard the ginger. Turn off the heat, and add one-quarter teaspoon of turmeric powder, one tablespoon of unflavored gelatin and one tablespoon of coconut oil. Stir until the gelatin is dissolved, then add one-half to one cup of calcium-enriched orange juice. Drink this tea once or twice a day.

Lydia Wilen and Joan Wilen are sisters who are folk-remedy experts based in New York City. The sisters are coauthors of many books, including *Bottom Line's Household Magic.*

Treat Gums to Ease Arthritis

P atients with rheumatoid arthritis and gum disease had tartar beneath gums scraped away so that gums could heal. After six weeks, patients had significantly less joint pain, stiffness and swelling. Patients whose gums were not treated did not improve. Reducing oral bacteria may ease inflammation elsewhere. See your dentist if gums bleed—and especially if joints ache, too.

Nabil Bissada, DDS, professor and chair, department of periodontics, Case Western Reserve University School of Dental Medicine, Cleveland, and leader of a study of 40 people.

Keep Your Hands Young and Strong—7 Simple Exercises Reduce Pain and Stiffness...In Just Minutes a Day

Anjum Lone, OTR/L, CHT, an occupational and certified hand therapist and chief of the department of occupational therapy at Phelps Memorial Hospital Center in Sleepy Hollow, New York.

If you have been diagnosed with arthritis, it's wise to protect your hands right away. Approximately 40% of arthritis patients must eventually restrict their daily activities because of joint pain or stiffness—and the hands often get the worst of it.

Both osteoarthritis (known as "wear-and-tear" arthritis) and rheumatoid arthritis (an autoimmune disease) can damage cartilage and sometimes the bones themselves.

What's missing from the typical arthritis prescription: Unfortunately, most patients with either type of arthritis do not recognize the importance of simple daily hand exercises, which can improve joint lubrication...increase your range of motion and hand strength...and maintain or restore function. These exercises also are helpful for people who have a hand injury or who heavily use their hands.

SAVE YOUR HANDS WITH EXERCISE

Most hand and wrist exercises can be done at home without equipment. But don't exercise during flare-ups, particularly if you have rheumatoid arthritis. Patients who ignore the pain and overuse their hands and wrists are more likely to suffer long-term damage, including joint deformity.

Important: Warm the joints before doing these exercises—this helps prevent microtears that can occur when stretching cold tissue. Simply run warm water over your hands in the sink for a few minutes right before the exercises. Or you can warm them with a heating pad.

Before doing the hand exercises here, it also helps to use the fingers of the other hand to rub and knead the area you'll be exercising.

This self-massage improves circulation to the area and reduces swelling.

If you have osteoarthritis or rheumatoid arthritis, do the following exercises five times on each hand—and work up to 10 times, if possible. The entire sequence should take no more than five minutes. Perform the sequence two to three times a day.*

• **Tendon glides.**

Purpose: Keeps the tendons functioning well to help move all the finger joints through their full range of motion.

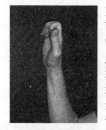

What to do: Rest your elbow on a table with your forearm and hand raised (fingertips pointed to the ceiling). Bend the fingers at the middle joint (form a hook with your fingers), and hold this position for a moment. Then bend the fingers into a fist, hiding your nails. Don't clench—just fold your fingers gently while keeping the wrist in a "neutral" position. Now make a modified fist with your nails showing. Next, raise your fingers so that they are bent at a 90-degree angle and your thumb is resting against your index finger (your hand will look similar to a bird's beak). Hold each position for three seconds.

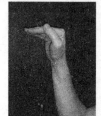

• **Thumb active range of motion.**

Purpose: Improves your ability to move your thumb in all directions. Do the movements gently so that you don't feel any pain.

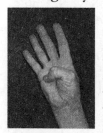

What to do: Rest your elbow on a table with your forearm and hand in the air. Touch the tip of the thumb to the tip of each finger (or get as close as you can). Then, flex the tip of your thumb toward the palm. Hold each of these positions for three seconds.

• **Web-space massage.**

Purpose: Using one hand to massage the other hand strengthens muscles in the "active"

*For more exercises, see an occupational therapist.

hand while increasing circulation in the "passive" hand.

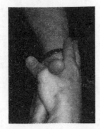

What to do: Clasp your left hand with your right hand as if you are shaking hands. With firm but gentle pressure, use the length of your left thumb to massage the web (space between the thumb and the index finger) next to your right thumb. Then, reverse the position and massage the web next to your left thumb. Massage each web for 30 seconds.

●**Wrist active range of motion.**

Purpose: To maintain proper positioning of the wrist, which helps keep the fingers in correct alignment.

What to do: Rest your right forearm on a table with your wrist hanging off the edge and your palm pointing downward—you'll only be

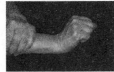

moving your wrist. Then place your left hand on top of your right forearm to keep it stable. With the fingers on your right hand held together gently, raise the wrist as high as it will comfortably go. Hold for three seconds.

Next, make a fist and raise it so the knuckles point upward. Now, lower the fist toward the floor. Hold each position for three seconds.

●**Digit extension.**

Purpose: Strengthens the muscles that pull the fingers straight—the movement prevents chronic contractions that can lead to joint deformity.

What to do: Warm up by placing the palms and fingers of both hands together and pressing the hands gently for five seconds. Then place your palms flat on a table. One at a time, raise each finger. Then lift all the fingers on one hand simultaneously while keeping your palm flat on the table. Hold each movement for five seconds.

●**Wrist flexion/extension.**

Purpose: Stretches and promotes muscle length in the forearm. Forearm muscles move the wrist and fingers. Flexion (bending your wrist so that your palm approaches the forearm) and extension (bending your wrist in the opposite direction) help maintain wrist strength and range of motion.

What to do: Hold your right hand in the air, palm down. Bend the wrist upward so that the tips of your fingers are pointed toward the

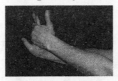

ceiling. Place your left hand against the fingers (on the palm side) and gently push so that the back of your right hand moves toward the top of your right forearm. Hold for 15 seconds. Switch hands and repeat.

Now, bend your right wrist downward so that the fingers are pointed at the floor. Place your left hand against the back of your right hand and gently push so your palm moves toward the bottom of the forearm. Hold 15 seconds. Switch and repeat.

●**Finger-walking exercises.**

Purpose: Strengthens fingers in the opposite direction of a deformity. This exercise is particularly helpful for rheumatoid arthritis patients.

What to do: Put one hand on a flat surface. Lift the index finger up and move it toward the thumb, then place the finger down. Next, lift the middle finger and move it toward the

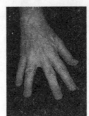

index finger. Lift the ring finger and move it toward the middle finger. Finally, lift the little finger and move it toward the ring finger. Repeat on your other hand.

Photos: Anjum Lone

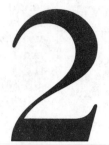

2

Emotional Health

Silence Your Inner Critic with Self-Compassion

Think of the last time you screwed something up. If you're like many women, your inner critic scolded, You're stupid, you're a loser, you don't deserve your job/friend/spouse/house. Then you probably bemoaned your lack of self-esteem and vowed to work harder to build it up—only to feel emotionally flattened again the next time you fell short.

That's because there is a problem with our repeated attempts to promote emotional health by inflating self-esteem, according to Kristin Neff, PhD, an associate professor in the educational psychology department at the University of Texas at Austin. "Our ultra-competitive culture tells us that we need to be constantly above average to feel good about ourselves—but there is always someone more successful, intelligent or attractive than we are. So we may wind up putting other people down in order to feel superior in comparison, which prevents us from seeing ourselves clearly and holds us back from reaching our full potential. And when we can't fool ourselves into believing that we're the best, we lose faith in ourselves and feel hopeless."

There is a better approach. Instead of trying to bolster self-esteem, Dr. Neff suggested building self-compassion—by learning to accept yourself with an open heart and treat yourself with the same kindness you would show to a friend.

Benefits: Studies link higher levels of self-compassion with greater life satisfaction, optimism, emotional intelligence and social connectedness...and less depression, anxiety and fear of failure.

Kristin Neff, PhD, associate professor of human development and culture in the educational psychology department at the University of Texas at Austin, and author of *Self-Compassion: Stop Beating Yourself Up and Leave Insecurity Behind.* She also is featured in the award-winning documentary and book *The Horse Boy,* a chronicle of her family's journey with autism. *Self-Compassion.org*

• **Self-compassion is not self-pity.** "Instead of emphasizing 'poor me,' the self-compassionate person recognizes that life is difficult for everyone," Dr. Neff explained. Nor is self-compassion an excuse for not even trying to do well. "Self-compassion motivates you to push through difficult challenges and to learn from your mistakes—without being devastated by them," she said.

PRACTICING THE ART OF SELF-COMPASSION

As with most things, self-compassion is a skill that improves with practice. In her book *Self-Compassion: Stop Beating Yourself Up and Leave Insecurity Behind,* Dr. Neff describes various exercises for learning to speak to yourself in a gentle and supportive manner. *Try the following techniques—at first you may feel silly, but soon you will see the benefits…*

• **Three-chair dialog.** Do this exercise whenever you are struggling with harsh self-judgment for a particular mistake or perceived character flaw. Place three empty chairs in a triangular configuration, several feet apart. Designate one chair for your inner self-critic…the second chair for the part of you that feels judged and criticized…and the third chair for a wise, compassionate observer. Now focus on the particular issue for which you are berating yourself.

Sit in the first chair and express out loud what your self-critic is thinking—for instance, *I hate it when you forget to pay the bills… you're so irresponsible.* Notice how that part of you is feeling—exasperated, self-righteous, worried.

Move to the second chair and express the thoughts of the criticized part of you—perhaps, *I feel hurt and overwhelmed, I'm too stressed to keep up with everything.* Notice what your body (slumped) and tone of voice (childlike, discouraged) seem to convey.

Continue the dialog between your self-critic and criticized self, physically moving from the first to the second chair and back again. Allow each part of yourself to express its views and be heard.

When you've exhausted the conversation, move to the third chair. In the role of observer, comment as wisely and compassionately as you can, as if offering insights to friends. You might say to the self-critic, *I see that you are worried and want to help prevent mistakes…*and to your criticized self, *It hurts to be judged harshly when you struggle with so many responsibilities and just want to be accepted for who you are.*

Review what you've learned from fully inhabiting both sides of yourself. Does your inner critic sound like your mother? Is "forgetting" to pay bills a form of rebellion? Keeping those insights in mind can help you remember to relate to yourself more kindly in the future.

• **Compassionate body scan.** This technique is particularly helpful when you are holding a lot of stress, physical discomfort or emotional pain in your body, Dr. Neff said. The point is to systematically focus attention on each area of your body, one part at a time, offering yourself compassion related to the problem in that area.

Lie on your back, arms at your sides, legs straight, feet shoulder-width apart and muscles relaxed. Starting at the top of your head, notice how your scalp feels. Is it itchy, tingling, hot? If there is discomfort, extend loving concern to that area by silently saying something like, *Poor darling, it will be OK, just relax.*

Move your focus to your face, then neck, then shoulders, etc., down to the soles of your feet, expressing compassion wherever you encounter aches or tension. This takes five to 30 minutes, depending on how you are feeling. For Dr. Neff's guided body scan, visit *www.self-compassion.org* and click on "Self-Compassion Practices (Guided Meditations and Exercises)."

• **Self-hug.** This can be done anytime you feel self-critical or upset. During particularly stressful periods, do it several times daily for at least a week.

Wrap your arms around yourself and give yourself a warm hug…gently rock your body… stroke your arms or face or put both hands gently over your heart…and focus on conveying self-love and tenderness.

In public, you can fold your arms and squeeze yourself gently or even just imagine hugging yourself comfortingly.

Why it works: Physical touch triggers release of oxytocin (called the hormone of love and bonding), calms cardiovascular stress and promotes a sense of security, Dr. Neff explained. That's why this simple technique is such a powerful way to build and express self-compassion.

Invite More Serenity Into Your Life

Judy Kuriansky, PhD, clinical psychologist and sex therapist on the adjunct faculty of Teachers College, Columbia University in New York City. She is the author of several books, including *The Complete Idiot's Guide to a Healthy Relationship*. DrJudy.com

Some people have a gift for staying serene even in circumstances that make others feel anxious and overwhelmed. This doesn't mean that they are overly passive—they just don't stress out over annoyances or waste energy trying to strong-arm situations that cannot be controlled. Their secret: They have discovered how to calm themselves in mind, body and spirit...so they're able to face life's challenges without getting frazzled or despondent.

Sounds wonderful, doesn't it? You don't have to be born with this talent. It's a skill that can be learned and refined. *Here's how…*

•**Give your mind a mini-vacation.** Mental chaos often results from overburdening yourself with responsibilities (think of your never-ending to-do list) or fretting about matters you cannot influence (the weather, the traffic, the economy).

What to do: When you feel such pressures mounting, remind yourself, *There's no need to think about this right now.* As simple as that sounds, it works. Then do something easy and pleasing—sing along with the radio, sort your lingerie drawer, soak in a warm bath—and feel the joy of focusing your attention only on this one activity, letting other thoughts float gently away. This calming technique is called mindfulness. Try it for a few minutes or an hour...or, ideally, indulge for an entire afternoon without ever checking the clock, telling yourself that you have all the time in the world.

•**Baby your body.** When you are over-stimulated, your heart races and adrenaline rushes through your body. In the short term, this keeps you alert and ready for action—but when it happens too often or too long, it leaves you feeling wired and decidedly unserene.

Whenever you feel the need to unwind physically: For several minutes, consciously move at half speed as you stroll around or do simple stretches...during this slow-motion respite, breathe deeply and luxuriate in the calming sensations seeping through your body. Physical touch is also extremely soothing, so take a few moments to stroke a pet or cuddle a soft pillow...smooth some lotion onto your skin...make gentle circles with your hand in the center of your chest...hug someone or ask a loved one to hug you.

•**Nurture your spirit.** Meditation is an excellent way to foster a sense of contentment and connection to your inner self and to the universe as a whole. Settle into a safe, quiet place...get into a comfortable position...then mentally visualize or gaze at a tranquil scene—a country landscape, a field of flowers, a starry sky.

Find it hard to sit still? Try a "moving meditation" by moving your body in flowing motions as you let your mind float freely...or, since water is calming, take a walk on a beach or alongside a pond. If it's consistent with your faith, recite the serenity prayer—God, grant me the serenity to accept the things I cannot change...the courage to change the things I can...and the wisdom to know the difference. This classic prayer has helped countless people fill their souls with a spirit of serenity.

Meditation Cuts Depression Symptoms Almost in Half

Sanford Nidich, EdD, associate director, Institute for Natural Medicine and Prevention at Maharishi University of Management in Fairfield, Iowa, and leader of two studies with a total of 112 people.

New research provides some good news about what is usually a sad topic—depression, a condition that not only obliterates joy but also contributes to cardiovascular disease. In two independent studies, researchers randomly assigned adults age 55 and older who had risk factors for cardiovascular disease to participate in a heart-healthy diet and exercise education group...or to practice Transcendental Meditation (TM) for 20 minutes twice per day. TM is a simple technique in which you silently repeat a mantra to let the mind settle down and reach a state of restful alertness. Participants were assessed with a standard test for depression over nine to 12 months.

Results: Compared with the education group, the TM group had significantly better scores on the depression test. The greatest improvement was seen among TM practitioners who had had significant depression at the start of the study—for them, depressive symptoms were reduced by 48%, on average. Implication: TM provides a double benefit, because preventing or easing depression also may reduce cardiovascular risk.

Editor's note: These studies looked specifically at TM, not at other meditation techniques, and were conducted by researchers at University of Hawaii, UCLA and Maharishi University of Management (which offers TM classes). For information on TM, visit *www.TM.org*... to learn about other meditation techniques, visit *www.How-To-Meditate.org.*

Reclaiming Your Life After Trauma

Judy Kuriansky, PhD, clinical psychologist and sex therapist on the adjunct faculty of Teachers College, Columbia University in New York City. She is the author of five books, including *The Complete Idiot's Guide to a Healthy Relationship.* DrJudy.com

You come home to find your house burglarized...your daughter has a serious car accident...you're laid off from a job you need and love...a friend loses her battle with cancer...or seemingly out of the blue, your husband demands a divorce. Such shocking and traumatic events wreak havoc with your emotions, leaving you struggling to pick up the pieces of your life. Nothing can make that task easy, but there are ways to make the challenge less daunting. *Here's what can help you cope after a trauma...*

•**Expect a myriad of reactions.** A disaster in your personal life inevitably triggers a range of reactions on many levels—emotional (panic, rage, desperation)...cognitive (confusion, indecision, obsessive thoughts)...physical (palpitations, breathlessness, insomnia, aches)... interpersonal (withdrawal, combativeness, distrustfulness)...and spiritual (questioning your faith or the meaning of life). Simply knowing that these experiences are normal can buffer their impact a bit.

•**Call yourself a survivor.** Of course, you did not choose for this traumatic event to occur, and it's understandable that you feel unjustly treated. But when you catch yourself thinking of yourself as a victim, try substituting the word survivor—you'll feel less helpless and more empowered.

•**Remember how you coped with past traumas.** Even if the current crisis is more severe than any difficulty you faced before, the coping techniques you used successfully in the past can be invaluable to you now. Do whatever makes you feel better—burn off anger in a fast-paced Zumba class, ease tension with a soothing bubble bath, find solace in the meditative repetition of weeding a garden. The stress that accompanies a crisis increases your risk for illness, so safeguard your health by eating well and getting to bed early. In talking with others, strive for balance—neither isolating yourself completely from friends and family nor obsessively repeating every detail of the trauma to anyone who's near. Reveal your feelings at your own pace, choosing trustworthy confidantes who listen empathically and help you process your experience and emotions.

●**Stay in the present.** There's no point in beating yourself up for a past event that you could not have foreseen or prevented ("If only I had told Aunt Trudy not to live in tornado country")...nor does it help to catastrophize about the future ("What if I never find another job and wind up on the streets?").

Better: Resume your normal daily activities to the extent possible...and take what comfort you can in small pleasures of the present moment. If you were to blame—for instance, you fell asleep at the wheel and caused an accident—you'll no doubt feel remorseful about what's past and must make whatever reparations you can, but try to focus mostly on learning lessons so you can prevent similar events in the future.

●**Consider professional help.** It is normal for a sense of loss to linger for a long time or to resurface on occasion (commonly on an anniversary). But it's best to see a counselor with expertise in bereavement or crisis counseling if you find it impossible to function...if extreme distress persists for more than a month...if people who know you well express concern about your behavior, appearance or well-being...or if you're tempted to "self-medicate" the pain away with excessive alcohol, pills or food or unsafe sexual activities. Get referrals from your doctor, insurance company and friends...or check online search engines for local grief therapists or counselors who treat post-traumatic stress disorder, then check out their credentials.

Let the crisis serve as a catalyst for change. Trauma provides an opportunity for reevaluating priorities. Decide what's truly important to you and take new directions accordingly—for instance, by finally pursuing your dream career, devoting more time to cherished relationships or embarking on a spiritual journey that will enrich the rest of your life.

The Six-Second Exercise that Short-Circuits Emotional Explosions

Marsha Lucas, PhD, is a licensed psychologist and neuropsychologist who has been studying the brain-behavior relationship for more than 20 years. She is the author of *Rewire Your Brain for Love: Creating Vibrant Relationships Using the Science of Mindfulness. Rewire YourBrainForLove.com*

W hat gets you spitting mad? A housemate leaving the sink full of dishes... a catty coworker's snide remarks...a fellow driver who cuts you off and then flips you the bird? It's understandable if such aggravations spark automatic angry outbursts—but blowing up may only make you feel worse.

There's a lightning-fast technique that helps calm emotional firestorms—a technique that takes a mere six seconds. According to neuropsychologist Marsha Lucas, PhD, author of the recent book *Rewire Your Brain for Love: Creating Vibrant Relationships Using the Science of Mindfulness*, this six-second method shares many similarities with mindfulness meditation, a practice where you simply notice your mind's busyness without getting carried away by it.

Why it works: Research shows that regularly practicing mindfulness meditation alters connections and pathways in the brain, actually changing the way the brain functions. For instance, meditation helps the prefrontal cortex (one of the main brain areas involved in thinking and impulse control) get better at detecting what's going on in the amygdala—the panic center where fear, anger and aggression are registered—and bathing that hair-trigger amygdala in soothing neurochemicals. In other words, Dr. Lucas explained, meditation develops a better "anger pause button," helping calm things down.

Similarly, with this six-second exercise, you consciously cultivate a habit of taking frequent mental pauses that allow your brain to "rest and restore." By practicing this technique throughout your day (not just when you're mad), you train your brain to pause automatically even in times of emotional upheaval. Thus, instead of getting hijacked by anger in the heat of the moment, you are able to make more mindful choices about how to react. As Dr. Lucas said, "You can put your foot on the brake—and not so hard that everyone with you gets whiplash."

What to do: The six-second technique takes longer to describe than to do, but it's very simple. *The steps…*

● **First, choose an external cue,** something that happens around 10 times a day—for example, turning on a faucet or checking your e-mail. Every time that cue occurs, use it as a reminder to do the exercise.

● **Silently say to yourself,** "My mind is alert, my body is calm," and inhale through your nose for a slow, easy count of three. Imagine your breath coming up from the bottoms of your feet and traveling through your legs, abdomen, chest, arms and shoulders…and invite a pleasant feeling of warmth to flow through your body.

● **Then exhale for a relaxed count of three (or even four),** letting your face, jaw and neck go loose. Allow that warm feeling to flow downward…imagine it carrying away any tension from your head, trunk and limbs and sending it out the bottoms of your feet. When you're done, gently resume your normal activity.

What to expect: With a regular practice of mindfulness, in a few weeks, you're likely to notice a reduction in angry fireworks…and a growing sense of emotional resilience, balance and calm.

Shop More, Live Longer

Yu-Hung Chang, PhD, is a researcher at the Institute of Population Health Sciences in Taiwan and leader of a study published in the *Journal of Epidemiology & Community Health*.

According to recent research, shopping is good for a person's health.

This study involved 1,841 seniors ages 65 and older who were asked how often they went shopping. Possible answers ranged from "daily" to "never."

Findings: Participants who reported shopping every day were 27% less likely to die during the study period than those who ventured out to stores less frequently.

Theory: Shopping involves various factors believed to extend longevity, including physical activity and increased social interaction.

Bottom line: Next time you feel the need for some retail therapy, don't feel guilty. You can even save your money—because window-shopping works, too.

The Link Between Sore Legs and Lingering Sadness

S. Marlene Grenon, MD, is an associate professor of surgery at the University of California, San Francisco, a vascular surgeon at the San Francisco VA Health Care System and lead author of an article on depression and PAD published in *Journal of the American Heart Association*.

The battle against depression is tough enough already without the added burden of physical illness. But unfortunately, depression can take a toll on the blood vessels…and a recent study has sounded a new note of caution about cardiovascular health.

We've known for a while that depression increases the risk for coronary artery disease, the narrowing of small blood vessels that supply blood and oxygen to the heart. But few studies have investigated a possible link between depression and peripheral artery disease (PAD), in which a buildup of plaque in the arteries reduces blood flow to the legs and feet. PAD patients often feel pain and fatigue in the leg or hip muscles when walking or climbing stairs...they also are vulnerable to hard-to-fight infections that can lead to gangrene. People with coronary artery disease are at especially high risk for PAD.

Researchers analyzed the records of 1,024 coronary artery disease patients, following the participants for an average of about seven years.

Findings: At the start of the study, PAD was seen in 12% of participants who were depressed but in only 7% of those who were not depressed. Similarly, by the end of the study, new problems with PAD had developed among 7% of depressed patients but only 5% of nondepressed participants.

The chicken or the egg? Researchers aren't sure which comes first, the PAD or the depression. Do PAD patients become depressed because they are in pain and aren't as mobile as they would like to be? Or do depressed people find it hard to summon the energy and motivation needed to follow a healthy lifestyle, which in turn increases their PAD risk? Or is it a vicious cycle, with each condition contributing to the other?

Whatever the connection, the researchers believe that healthy habits—including a good diet, regular exercise, weight control, smoking avoidance and stress management—may improve both PAD and depression. So if you're struggling with either ailment, talk to your doctor about the lifestyle and treatment options that can help you feel your best...both physically and emotionally.

All Women Are Beautiful When They Dance

Sarah Hiner, president of the Bottom Line family of newsletters and books... and competitive ballroom dancer. Follow Hiner on Twitter: @SarahHiner

Dancing is great exercise, of course, with proven physical health benefits such as improved balance, endurance, strength, agility, flexibility and cardiovascular fitness.

But ballroom dancing in particular provides a bonus benefit that keeps women coming back for more: No matter what their size or shape, the act of ballroom dancing makes all women feel elegant and beautiful. When competing, women don sparkling dresses, fancy hairstyles and dazzling make-up that take even the most ordinary-looking women and make them feel like swans.

To find ballroom dancing classes in your area, check your local newspapers or phone directories. There are national franchises, such as Fred Astaire (*www.fredastaire.com*) and Arthur Murray (*www.arthurmurray.com*), as well as smaller independent studios. Most dance studios allow prospective students to take a test lesson before signing up for classes. Instructors come in all levels of skill and experience, so be sure that you find an instructor who makes you feel comfortable—since your bodies will be touching. As you improve, you may move on to other classes and other instructors.

Even beginners can participate in competitions with other novices, which is very fun and glamorous—but it's not necessary to compete to enjoy yourself. I compete occasionally, but primarily I dance because each week it provides a little romantic vacation from my hectic life. So whether or not you compete, you can feel as magically transformed as Cinderella at the ball.

Belt Out a Song for Better Health

Michael Miller, MD, is a professor of medicine, epidemiology and preventive medicine at the University of Maryland School of Medicine and director of the Center for Preventive Cardiology for the University of Maryland Medical System, both in Baltimore. He is a past president of the American Society of Preventive Cardiology and has been listed among the "Most Influential Doctors" (*USA Today*), "Super Doctors" (*Washington Post Magazine*) and *"America's Top Doctors"* (Castle Connolly).

Opening our mouths for a bite of the proverbial "apple a day" has its place—but to really keep the doctor away, we should open wide and let out some songs. Why? Because singing has numerous health benefits, recent research shows. And the rewards are ours even if we warble off-key or forget half the lyrics.

We spoke with Michael Miller, MD, director of the Center for Preventive Cardiology for the University of Maryland Medical System, who has researched music's health effects, to discuss the specifics. He pointed out that singing's positive effects are both psychological and physical. *For instance, bursting into song can…*

•**Make you happier and more relaxed.** It boosts production of the feel-good brain chemicals called endorphins…and reduces blood levels of the stress hormone cortisol that is associated with anxiety and depression. Singing also encourages a breathing pattern—with a shorter inhalation and longer exhalation—that promotes relaxation. What's more, songs with personal significance can help you recall positive memories and emotions.

•**Promote cardiovascular health.** Again, endorphins get the credit—because their release causes blood vessels to dilate, allowing blood to flow more easily and reducing blood pressure, Dr. Miller said. For best effect, choose joyful songs, not mournful tunes.

•**Provide aerobic and respiratory benefits.** Singing requires you to take deep breaths. This increases levels of oxygen in the bloodstream, promoting mental alertness…helps clear respiratory tubes and sinuses…and increases your lung capacity.

•**Build strength.** The muscles of your chest, abdomen, back and face all get a workout when you sing your heart out.

How much should you sing? The more the better! *To mix more melody-making into your day…*

•**Think of the world as your stage.** You can croon just about anywhere—not only in the bathroom as you shower, but also in the kitchen while you're cooking, in the car on your way to work or wherever else the urge strikes.

•**Be a songwriter.** Don't worry if you can't remember the words to your favorite songs. Exercise your creativity by making up your own lyrics…or just sing nonsense syllables for the fun of it.

•**Join a musical group.** This has the advantage of assuring that singing becomes part of your regular schedule, and it may lead to new friendships and an increased sense of community. So check out the opportunities with a local musical theater troupe, church choir or amateur band.

•**Try karaoke.** Many karaoke machines for home use are available at electronics stores, mass merchandisers and online. To check out some options, visit *www.KaraokeMachine Reviews.org*. When you're ready to go public, Google "karaoke" plus the name of your town to find local venues that host karaoke nights.

•**Go "caroling"—any time of year.** Who says that door-to-door songfests can occur only during December? Gather up family or friends and spread some melodic merriment throughout your neighborhood. Or take your group to a nearby nursing home to lead a sing-along with the residents—helping to boost their health and mood as well as your own.

How to Finally Forgive Yourself...and Move Forward

Fred Luskin, PhD, director of the Stanford University Forgiveness Projects and professor of clinical psychology at Sofia University in Palo Alto, California. He is author of *Forgive for Love. LearningToForgive.com*

Women tend to be hard on themselves, turning isolated errors into cause for sweeping self-condemnation. *I failed at that task* becomes *I am a failure...I gained a few pounds* becomes *I'm fat and ugly...I hurt someone I love* becomes *I'm a terrible wife.* This often makes it difficult for women to forgive themselves for their mistakes and shortcomings. Fortunately, research has revealed proven techniques that help people pardon themselves.

Why make the effort: Self-forgiveness can lead to improved health, reduced stress, better relationships, personal growth and inner peace. *Steps to take...*

•**Identify your "grievance story."** This is the story that replays in your mind, focusing on your flaws. Write it down...then consider how you vilify yourself.

Example: "My best friend dumped me because I'm clingy and controlling. I deserve to be lonely." Now rewrite this as a "forgiveness story" by emphasizing good intentions and lessons learned—"What I did was done out of love...but now I see that people need space and I'm working to improve my relationships."

•**Challenge unenforceable rules.** Make a list of the rules or beliefs you judge yourself by—that loving mothers don't lose their tempers, that you must always make wise financial decisions.

Ask: "Is it possible for me—or anyone—to adhere to such rules?" If not, change your rules to conform to the reality that people do frequently fail. Doing your best doesn't require perfection.

•**Label your dreams.** A big dream is to find a fulfilling career or a loving lifelong companion...a small dream is that a particular job or a particular romantic relationship is "the one." Failing at a small dream does not doom the big dream. Make a course correction if necessary (for instance, by acknowledging that a career in sales or a long-distance relationship is not right for you), then keep moving toward the real goal—your big dream.

•**Make amends.** We've all been hurtful at one time or another...but making amends allows you to make peace with the past.

What to do: Sincerely apologize to, and practice kindness toward, the people you wronged. If they are not available, use symbolic acts of kindness.

Examples: Volunteer in a nursing home if you blame yourself for not having helped your elderly parents enough...give money to charity if you fudged on your taxes. Even if someone you harmed won't forgive you, trying to make amends helps you forgive yourself.

Tap Away Fears and Phobias

Shoshana Garfield, PhD, psychologist, Registered Trauma Specialist and CEO and Head of Training and Coaching, Dance Tree Solutions. *UnlimitedEmotional Freedom.com*

There is a fascinating method that may help melt away fears and phobias. Called Thought Field Therapy (TFT), the technique is designed to help people permanently free themselves from phobias (strong, irrational fears of things that pose little or no actual danger), such as fear of spiders or of public speaking...and even from post-traumatic stress disorder (PTSD), an anxiety disorder that can develop after a terrifying event in which grave harm occurred or was threatened. No medications are used, so there are no side effects. TFT falls within the field of energy psychology. TFT involves thinking about the feared object or event while tapping specific points on the face and body and humming, counting or moving the eyes.

Since TFT sounded almost too good to be true, we interviewed psychologist Shoshana Garfield, PhD, who uses TFT to help patients overcome phobias and PTSD. She said that TFT has roots in acupuncture, in that you tap on points that correspond to energy meridians. This helps unblock the body's energy system, which can become overwhelmed by fear, Dr. Garfield said. TFT also simultaneously provides sensory data to the right brain (the emotional side) and left brain (the logical side). This stimulates activity of both brain hemispheres and of the corpus callosum that connects them…deactivates signals associated with fear-triggered hyperarousal of the limbic system…and "rewires" cognitive function, releasing distress.

Evidence: In a 2010 study, PTSD patients treated with TFT showed dramatic decreases in nightmares, flashbacks, concentration problems, jumpiness, aggression and isolation. Other studies have demonstrated TFT's effectiveness in reducing depression…and in patients with anxiety disorder, EEG scans showed that abnormal brain wave patterns associated with anxiety normalized after TFT treatment.

Citing the classic example from TFT founder Roger Callahan, PhD, Dr. Garfield described a woman who had a lifelong fear of water. After more than a year of ineffective conventional treatment, Dr. Callahan instructed the woman to tap a spot under each eye while looking at a swimming pool. After a few minutes of tapping, she said that she no longer felt any fear, then ran to the pool and splashed water on her face—something she could not do previously.

TRYING TFT FOR YOURSELF

For best results, Dr. Garfield recommended working with a psychologist trained in TFT who can provide testimonials from other patients with phobias similar to yours.

Referrals: Association for Comprehensive Energy Psychology (visit *www.energypsych. org* and click on "membership" and then "member directory")…or Association for the Advancement of Meridian Energy Techniques (visit *www.aamet.org* and click on "search for members")…or Dr. Roger Callahan (*http://tft tapping.com*). Results might be seen after just

one treatment for a simple phobia or might take nine months or longer for PTSD. Are you skeptical? That's OK—because TFT works even if you don't believe in it, Dr. Garfield noted.

For simple fears that are not deeply interwoven with complex traumas, you may find relief on your own with the tapping sequence below. Practice it several times until you know the steps…then do the sequence whenever you anticipate or encounter the feared object or event. (Use common sense, of course—for instance, by tapping before you get behind the wheel, rather than while you are driving.) The routine takes just a few minutes and, though it may seem complicated at first, it soon becomes second nature, Dr. Garfield said.

Demo: *www.youtube.com/watch?v=ntWUsL 5bZJ0.*

Step 1: Focus attention on the thing you fear. For instance, visualize a spider or imagine driving through a construction zone. Important: Keep thinking about the object of your fear throughout your TFT session.

Step 2: Rate your fear level on a scale of zero to 10. Zero would indicate no distress whatsoever and 10 would be the worst it could possibly be. Remember this number.

Step 3: Tap. Use the tips of the index and middle fingers of either hand to tap firmly (but not hard enough to hurt) five to 10 times, at a moderately fast pace. First tap four inches below either armpit (about at the center of the band on your bra)…then tap one inch below the center of either eye.

Step 4: Perform the nine-step "gamut sequence." Make a loose fist with your nondominant hand and locate what TFT practitioners call the gamut spot on the back of that hand, in the hollow an inch below the knuckles of the ring and little fingers. Start tapping this gamut spot with the index and middle fingers of your dominant hand.

Continuing tapping, giving five to 10 taps for each of the following actions.

Gamut sequence: Open eyes wide…close eyes…open eyes and (keeping head still) look down and to the left…look down and to the right…roll eyes around counterclockwise…roll eyes around clockwise…hum a few bars of any song (activating the right brain)…count aloud from one to five (activating the left brain)… hum again. When finished, repeat the gamut sequence a second time.

Step 5: Rate your fear again, from zero to 10. If your score has dropped to zero, terrific! If it has not, repeat all the TFT steps one or more times, continuing to visualize the object of your phobia. Then, again rate your fear level—which may now be much lower.

Smile! Even a Fake Grin Is Good for You

Sarah D. Pressman, PhD, associate professor of psychology and social behavior at the University of California, Irvine and coauthor of a study on facial expression and stress in *Psychological Science.*

Can't get the checkbook to balance? Stubbed your toe so hard you see stars? You may feel like cursing or crying…but try forcing a smile instead. You'll be surprised at how this can help both your mood and your health when you're struggling with a stressful situation, whether the challenge is psychological or physical. And don't worry if that smile isn't sincere—because even a fake one will do the trick, a recent study reveals.

To understand the new research, first envision these two different types of smiles: A "standard" smile involves only the muscles of the mouth…in contrast, a genuine smile involves the mouth muscles as well the muscles around the eyes. (It makes sense—think about how much a pair of twinkly, crinkly eyes contributes to a truly happy facial expression.)

For the study, all participants had to complete two stressful tasks. First they were instructed to spend two minutes tracing a star with their nondominant hands (the left hand for most people) while being able to see only a reflection of the star and hand in a mirror. For the second task, they had to keep their hands submerged in ice water for one minute.

What differed were the facial expressions that participants were instructed to maintain throughout the tasks. One group maintained a neutral expression…another group kept a standard mouth-only smile on their faces…a third group did its best to have a genuine crinkly-eyed smile. To ensure that the assigned expression was produced, each participant was trained to hold chopsticks in his or her mouth in a specific way designed to engage the appropriate facial muscles. In addition, in the standard smile and genuine smile groups, half of the participants were specifically asked to smile during the tasks, while the other half were given no particular instructions about smiling.

Before, during and for some minutes after each task, researchers recorded each participant's heart rate.

Reason: The heart speeds up in times of stress…and the rate at which it slows back down and recovers is linked to future heart-health outcomes. Participants also were questioned about their perceived levels of stress.

Results: Compared with the nonsmilers, the groups that smiled during the stressful tasks—whether or not they were consciously aware of and trying to grin—had faster heart-rate recovery times after the tasks and lower self-reported levels of stress. Those with genuine smiles that reached the eyes had a slight advantage, but even those who smiled only with their mouths were less stressed than those who didn't smile at all.

Explanation? Researchers hypothesize that activating the facial muscles involved in smiling can stimulate certain brain regions associated with positive emotions, thus triggering those emotions and reducing the intensity of the body's stress response.

How this info can help you: When faced with some stressful physical or psychological unpleasantness such as getting an injection, being stuck in traffic or struggling with a tough task at work, remember that "grin and bear it" is good advice—especially the grin part—benefiting both your mood and your heart.

Phone Therapy Can Be Effective

David C. Mohr, PhD, director, Center for Behavioral Intervention Technologies and professor of preventive medicine, Feinberg School of Medicine, Northwestern University, Chicago.

Researchers recently analyzed 12 studies on psychotherapy for adults that was conducted by telephone and involved at least four sessions (typically 45 to 50 minutes each).

Result: About 8% of patients discontinued treatment soon after its start compared with an average dropout rate of nearly 47% for those receiving traditional face-to-face psychotherapy. Telephone therapy also appeared to be as effective at treating depression as office visits.

Theory: Telephone psychotherapy transcends barriers to office sessions, such as transportation problems or juggling appointments with work and family obligations. Anyone who is considering discontinuing psychotherapy treatments because of time constraints or transportation problems should ask his/her therapist if phone therapy is an option.

Who Could Develop a Drinking Problem?

Stephanie Brown, PhD, a licensed psychologist and director of the Addictions Institute in Menlo Park, California. She also is the author of many books on addiction and recovery and was the founder of the Alcohol Clinic at Stanford University Medical Center in Stanford, California.

It's heartbreaking to watch a loved one slide down that slippery slope from social drinking to problem drinking to alcoholism—or to slide down it yourself. But did you know that this can happen to almost anyone, at almost any point in life? And women in midlife or beyond are certainly not immune.

But: Because many people do not realize this, it is easy for an older woman's descent into addiction to go unrecognized until the problem is very advanced...or until a tragedy occurs.

Psychologist Stephanie Brown, PhD, director of the Addictions Institute in Menlo Park, California, explained, "Aging brings new and different stresses that may cause a woman to turn to alcohol even if she did not do so in the past."

Examples: In midlife, a woman may feel lonely when children leave home...disappointed if a career stalls...strained by providing care for elderly parents...or adrift if a marriage ends in divorce. Later in life, she may experience a sense of purposelessness or financial insecurity after retirement...anxiety about health problems...or grief when loved ones pass away.

Certain physiological factors of aging also contribute to a woman's risk, according to the book *Women Under the Influence* from the National Center on Addiction and Substance Abuse (CASA) at Columbia University. Physical tolerance for alcohol diminishes as her lean muscle mass ebbs, metabolism slows, and liver and kidney function decline. This leaves an older woman with a higher blood alcohol level than a younger woman who drinks the same amount.

Consequence: A level of drinking that appeared to be safe and moderate in earlier adulthood can become addicting as the years pass.

Some research has shown that women experience higher rates of late-onset alcoholism than men do, the CASA researchers reported, perhaps due to higher rates of stress. About half of all cases of alcoholism among older women begin after age 59—compared with only one-fourth of cases among older men.

HOW ALCOHOL SUCKS WOMEN IN

A mature woman who honed her natural coping skills as a younger adult may be less likely to develop an alcohol problem than one who sometimes relied on outside substances to relieve stress. But even a woman who usually copes well can slide into abuse.

Dr. Brown explained, "It's subtle, but sometimes a person just begins to turn toward alcohol. For instance, a woman accustomed to a daily glass of wine might notice that having a little more helps her feel better. She thinks, So what's a little more?" Gradually the habit grows...until it is much more than a habit.

An alcoholic is drawn to alcohol the way a person is drawn to a lover—she feels excited when they are together and wants that experience every day. Once that love is established, the alcoholic makes lifestyle changes that allow her to drink more. She may socialize only with friends who enjoy drinking...bring wine to a party as a "gift" or carry little bottles in her purse to ensure that alcohol is available...or spend increasing amounts of time drinking alone at home. Despite this, she may insist that she does not have a drinking problem—because denial is a common characteristic of addiction.

Meanwhile, people around her may fail to recognize the situation.

Reasons: An older woman's drinking is less obviously disruptive to the family than it is when young children live at home. Doctors often neglect to screen older women for alcoholism—according to CASA researchers, only 17% of female patients age 65 and over said that their doctors asked about alcohol during a checkup. And when possible symptoms of alcohol abuse (memory problems, fatigue, headache, insomnia) are present, older women often are misdiagnosed with depression, anxiety or age-related cognitive decline.

Result: Among the estimated two million American women over age 59 who might benefit from treatment for alcohol abuse, less than 1% receive such treatment.

SPOTTING THE WARNING SIGNS

Moderate drinking for women typically is defined as no more than one serving of alcohol per day—that's 12 ounces of beer, five ounces of wine or 1.5 ounces of liquor. But people in denial about their drinking may dismiss that limit as absurdly strict. Often this denial continues until—or even after—they pass out at a party, get arrested for drunk driving, wake up in a stranger's bed or cause a serious accident.

But quantity doesn't tell the whole story. Dr. Brown said, "Getting hooked psychologically is independent from the quantity of alcohol consumed. If that one drink per day becomes the focus of a person's life or if she feels like she cannot enjoy dinner without a drink, that is a warning of psychological dependence."

Reason: The defining characteristic of addiction is loss of control—over when you drink...or how much you drink...or the way in which you think about drinking.

Bottom line: A woman should seek help from her doctor or a therapist if she frequently drinks more often or in greater quantity than she intended...or if she experiences cravings for or obsessive thoughts about alcohol. Does this describe you or a loved one? Remember that there is always hope—because just as a woman is never too old to develop a drinking problem, she is never too old to recover.

How to Love Life Again After Losing a Spouse

Becky Aikman, a New York–based journalist and author of *Saturday Night Widows: The Adventures of Six Friends Remaking Their Lives*, the memoir of a group that Aikman founded to help herself and five other widows focus on happiness rather than grief. The former *BusinessWeek* editor lost her husband to cancer in 2004 after 20 years of marriage. *BeckyAikman.com*

Becky Aikman was in her 40s when she lost her husband to cancer. She formed a group with five other widows.

Their goal: To learn to live again after the worst thing that ever happened to them.

In the process, they found that some of the traditional thinking about loss and recovery wasn't helpful.

Here, advice for rebuilding your life—when you feel ready to do so—in the months or years after the death of your husband or wife...

AVOID COMMON TRAPS

Beware the missteps that can stand in the way of remaking your life.

•**Don't put off rebuilding because you haven't yet experienced the stages of grief.** In the late 1960s, a psychiatrist named Elisabeth

Kübler-Ross popularized the idea that the grieving process has five predictable stages—denial, anger, bargaining, depression and acceptance. These "five stages of grief" have become so ingrained in our culture that some widows and widowers believe they can't be truly ready to move on with their lives if they haven't yet passed through each of them. In fact, these stages were never intended to apply to grieving spouses but only to those who were dying themselves.

People who lose a spouse often experience waves of emotion separated by periods of feeling relatively normal. Over time, the waves become less extreme and less frequent until the widow or widower feels ready to reengage with humanity.

● **Be wary of support groups.** These groups are supposed to help widows and widowers cope with their grief by talking about it with others. Trouble is, spending time with other grieving people and focusing your attention on your grief can make you sadder.

Give one of these groups a try if you think talking about your grief might help. But if you discover that it isn't for you, don't feel that your recovery depends on your continued attendance.

● **Make decisions based on what you want your life to look like in the future, not on maintaining the life you had before.** It can be very difficult to give up the plans we made with our late partners, but those plans might no longer be appropriate for us.

Example: Some widows hang onto the family home, even though they no longer need the space, and then feel isolated living in communities full of families. Many who move into smaller homes closer to other singles are glad they did.

FRIENDS

It might make sense to alter whom you socialize with or how you arrange to spend time with them…

● **Be proactive about making plans with friends.** You can't just sit at home waiting for friends to call with things for you to do. Your friends might go out of their way to extend invitations in the months immediately after your spouse passes away, but those invitations are likely to eventually dry up as your friends return to their normal patterns and forget that you're sitting home alone. It's up to you to contact them to make plans. Do this days or weeks in advance, when possible, to reduce the odds that they already will have made plans.

● **Construct a new circle of single friends.** If you and your late spouse were like most married couples, you probably socialized mainly with other married couples. You might start to feel like a fifth wheel if couples remain your only friends. If other members of your circle have also lost their spouses, make a particular effort to socialize with them. If you don't have unattached friends, ask your friends if they have other friends who have lost their partners or are otherwise unmarried and suggest that they be invited to get-togethers, too.

● **Get over any guilt about new romantic relationships.** Widows and widowers often worry that seeing someone new implies that their departed spouse wasn't really the love of their life. This isn't true—researchers have found that it's people who were very deeply in love with their departed spouses who are most likely to find love again.

ACTIVITIES

Certain pursuits are particularly worthwhile when you're trying to recover from the loss of a spouse.

● **Seek new experiences.** Explore new hobbies. Visit new places. Take classes in subjects you know little about.

Examples: I attended the opera, took architecture tours and joined a group of friends on a spa trip, all things I don't normally do.

Doing new things isn't just enjoyable—it also helps widows and widowers gain confidence in their ability to face new challenges. That can be very empowering for people worried that they might not have it in them to remake their lives after decades of marriage and routine.

● **Cook well for yourself.** Losing a spouse can mean losing the person who cooked for you…or losing the person for whom you cooked. Either way, the result often is a dramatic decline in the quality of the surviving spouse's meals. (When the survivor is the cook, he/she often concludes that it isn't worth preparing elaborate meals that no one else will eat.)

Dining out can be challenging, too. Many newly widowed people find it uncomfortable and boring to eat alone in restaurants.

But if you stop eating well after the loss of a spouse, you deny yourself an important source of pleasure when you need it most. Your health might suffer, too, if you resort to junk food.

What to do: Make cooking good food a priority, even if you're the only one who will eat it. If your late spouse was the cook in the family, enroll in cooking classes. Not only can these classes teach you to cook well for yourself, but you also might meet new friends.

•**Travel with tour groups.** Travel is an excellent way to have new and enjoyable experiences, but many people find it awkward to travel alone, and not having someone to share travel experiences with can detract from the fun.

If you travel with a tour group, you'll have people with whom you can share the adventure. You might even form lasting friendships with other members of the group.

Helpful: Before signing up for a trip, call the tour operator to confirm that a significant number of the members of the group are single. It can be uncomfortable to be the only one traveling alone in a group.

Family Peace Hidden In Family Photos

Barbara Okun, PhD, coauthor of *Saying Goodbye: How Families Can Find Renewal Through Loss.*

When viewed in a particular way, family photos not only can help you bear the grief when a loved one is close to death or has recently died, they also can help you mend strained relationships with family members who remain.

The secret: Create a family photo biography, a sort of visual family timeline.

Barbara Okun, PhD, a clinical psychologist/family therapist and coauthor of *Saying Goodbye: How Families Can Find Renewal Through Loss*, said that, in addition to keeping treasured memories alive and fostering introspection that leads to personal growth, a photo biography can help you resolve long-standing grievances and misunderstandings. Why bother unearthing long-buried family issues at this point? "Because these issues will emerge, and they will affect the way the family responds to the crisis of a relative's terminal diagnosis or death. To prevent them from further poisoning the waters, it is better to identify and face unresolved grievances now, and really put them to rest, instead of thinking you can sweep them under the carpet," she said.

How to make your family's photo biography: Start by assembling a collection of family photos spanning as many years as possible, Dr. Okun advised. Look through your old photo albums and computer photo files…check archived images on Facebook and print the ones you want to include…ask relatives and friends to contribute photos, too. The idea is to compile a mix of old and new photos of your loved one, yourself and your other immediate and extended family members. Aim for at least one dozen to two dozen photos.

Clear a large tabletop so you have plenty of space to work—this has the advantage of allowing you to see all your photos at once. Arrange the photos in chronological order, starting with the oldest photos at the top of the table and ending with the newest ones at the bottom.

Now, study the pictures to see what memories, feelings, questions and concerns they might evoke. Ponder your place in the family…your relationship with the person who is ill or whose loss you are mourning…and the connections between you and the other members of your family. *To get started on this introspection, ask yourself questions such as…*

• **What memories are being most powerfully triggered as I look at the photos of my loved one?** What emotions surface for me as I contemplate these memories?

• **How have my feelings toward this person changed over time, and what precipitated those changes?** What regrets do I have about my relationship with my loved one? What would I change if I could, or what can I do now to mend the relationship?

• **Am I jealous of, angry with or emotionally distant from any other family member now, and how does that make me feel?** If that person were dying, would my feelings about our strained relationship change?

• **To whom in the family am I closest now, and to whom was I closest in the past?** Am I content with the current level of closeness? Is there anything I'd like to do to be even closer?

As you study the photos: Look for patterns in relationships that are no longer serving you well. For instance, the photos may remind you of the way your older brother always took charge when you were growing up—but now you realize that you don't want him to make all the decisions during the current crisis of a parent's decline.

Also take note of anything that surprises you. For instance, do you see an unexpectedly vulnerable or tender expression on the face of the sister whom you always considered hard-hearted? Are there a surprising number of photos of your "workaholic" father playing ball or clowning around with you? Such concrete evidence may convince you that distorted memories have been detrimental to your relationships.

If you realize that you regret a rift with a loved one who has already died, you can still make some peace with the past. For instance, try writing that person a letter or imagining a detailed conversation in your head, saying whatever you wish you had said while the person was still alive. Then imagine yourself forgiving yourself for your part of the conflict.

If you realize that you want a closer relationship with a family member who's still alive, don't be afraid to reach out to that person and explain how you're feeling…while there's still

time to mend fences. How to open that conversation? "You can say, 'I'm feeling bad about the rupture in our relationship. I would like to hear your thoughts and feelings about it and take responsibility for my part.' Or sometimes asking another relative to initiate the contact can be helpful," Dr. Okun suggested. "The point is that all parties to a relationship bear some responsibility for that relationship, both positive and negative. It takes both parties to reconcile—so if the other party does not want to engage with you, at least you know you tried."

Mourning the Loss of a Beloved Pet

Alan D. Wolfelt, PhD, is a psychologist, founder and director of the Center for Loss & Life Transition in Fort Collins, Colorado. He is the author of more than 25 books on grief and loss, including *When Your Pet Dies: A Guide to Mourning, Remembering and Healing. CenterForLoss.com

It is not at all silly—or uncommon—to feel overwhelmed with sorrow when a beloved pet passes away, given that many pet owners consider their dogs, cats and other lovable critters to be members of the family. Yet because some people regard a pet as "just an animal," they may not offer appropriate emotional support (as they would if you had lost a relative, for instance)—and the lack of understanding makes it harder to get through this difficult time. You may even doubt the legitimacy of your grief, believing it to be excessive, which also stymies attempts to mourn and move on.

We spoke with psychologist and grief counselor Alan D. Wolfelt, PhD, author of *When Your Pet Dies: A Guide to Mourning, Remembering, and Healing*, to discuss ways to ease the pain after the loss of a pet. *His suggestions…*

• **Recognize the depth of your grief as a reflection of the strength of your love and depth of relationship.** "The more profound the attachment to your pet was, the more profound your grief is likely to be," Dr. Wolfelt said.

• **Accept that all your feelings are valid.** Along with sadness, you may experience a surprising array of emotions—anger, denial, confusion, relief (if the animal had been suffering), even guilt (if you euthanized your pet or were unable to keep it safe from harm). These feelings are normal.

• **Seek support from other pet lovers.** Friends and relatives who care as deeply for their animals as you did for yours can sympathize, understanding the bond you shared with your pet.

Also helpful: Pet grief support groups. Ask your veterinarian for a referral to a local group…or check *www.pet-loss.net.*

• **Express your grief.** Write in a journal, compose a song, paint or sculpt—any activity into which you can pour your grief helps you process painful emotions, said Dr. Wolfelt.

• **Consider whether there is a deeper well of pain within you.** If you seem stuck in your grief, perhaps losing your pet triggered a subconscious review of an earlier loss. Dr. Wolfelt explained, "You may not have mourned adequately for a previous death—for instance, of a parent. The pet's death can bring out those repressed feelings, making your current grief seem out of proportion." If you suspect this, consult a therapist or grief counselor for help in finally mourning your earlier loss.

• **Create a ritual to honor your pet.** Having a funeral or memorial service for your pet encourages family members to openly express their emotions, formally acknowledge the loss and share comforting memories.

Also helpful: Create a scrapbook dedicated to your pet, with photos and small mementos such as a collar tag.

• **Think carefully before getting a new pet.** The decision about whether or when to acquire another animal is highly individual, so only you can say when you're ready.

But: If you bring another pet into your home before you have truly accepted that your previous companion is gone and cannot be replaced, you may be disappointed. As Dr. Wolfelt said, "First you must allow yourself to mourn the death of your pet—because that is what lets you open your heart to the love and companionship a new pet can provide."

3

Ease Fibromyalgia, Chronic Fatigue and More...

Fibromyalgia Breakthrough: Unlearn Your Pain

Fibromyalgia affects an estimated 5 million Americans (most of them middle-aged women)—and is a very mysterious and frustrating disorder, for people with the condition and professionals who try to treat it.

"People diagnosed with fibromyalgia have pain throughout their bodies, usually in a dozen or more 'tender points' in muscles—but no one can tell them why," says Howard Schubiner, MD, director of the Mind-Body Medicine Center of the St. John Providence Health System in Warren, Michigan, and author of *Unlearn Your Pain* (MindBody Publishing).

"There's no actual tissue breakdown or destruction—nothing conventionally 'wrong' in the muscles, tendons, joints or bones," he continues. "But brain imaging studies show that the pain and suffering is real, and is felt in much the same way a person feels a broken bone. And like a broken bone, the pain of fibromyalgia can be severe and even debilitating, forcing a person to spend days in bed."

And that's not the only problem. According to Dr. Schubiner, people with fibromyalgia commonly have other health problems, such as lower back pain, migraine or tension headaches, jaw and face pain from temporomandibular joint disorder, bowel and bladder syndromes, and insomnia.

"Needless to say, it's very frustrating for a person with widespread pain to have no idea what is causing it, and to be considered crazy by some and incurable by others—and to get little or no relief from pain medications, muscle relaxants, antidepressants and mood stabilizers," Dr. Schubiner says.

But now there is relief from fibromyalgia—without drugs.

Howard Schubiner, MD, director of the Mind-Body Medicine Center of the St. John Providence Health System in Warren, Michigan, and is author of *Unlearn Your Pain*.

Striking research finding: A study by Dr. Schubiner and his colleagues in the *Journal of Internal Medicine* shows that a focus on the pain-triggering role of negative emotions and stress in fibromyalgia can dramatically reduce pain—and even clear up the condition!

THE STRESS–PAIN CONNECTION

The researchers studied 45 middle-aged women who had been suffering from fibromyalgia for an average of 13 years.

The women were divided into two groups. One group received four weeks of a therapy called Affective Self-Awareness (ASA)—learning about and accepting the connection between emotions, stress, and the pain of fibromyalgia and learning and practicing techniques for expressing and releasing emotions and reducing stress. The other group was put on a waiting list to receive ASA. Pain levels were measured at the start of the study and six months later.

After six months, pain had been eliminated or reduced to very low levels in 25% of the ASA group—in effect, their fibromyalgia had gone into remission. Overall, nearly half of the ASA group had pain reduction of 30% or more.

"These results may not seem remarkable," says Dr. Schubiner. "But consider this—these reductions in pain were measured at six months and are therefore long-lasting, and they are greater than the results found in studies of medications for fibromyalgia. In fact, the women in the wait-listed group were using medications for fibromyalgia during the six months of the study—and had no reduction in pain."

Why it works: Fibromyalgia pain is real, emphasizes Dr. Schubiner. It is processed through the central nervous system along "learned nerve pathways" that are created and then repeatedly triggered by emotional trauma and stress—in exactly the same way you create nerve pathways when you learn to ride a bicycle and then use those same pathways for the rest of your life whenever you ride a bike. Sometimes the origin of the trauma and stress—the "priming" event that sets you up for fibromyalgia—is in childhood (for example, physical or sexual abuse, the death of a parent).

Sometimes the priming event is in adulthood (for example, marital difficulties, problems at work).

Fact: Over half of people with fibromyalgia have post-traumatic stress disorder (PTSD) or PTSD-like symptoms, such as depression and anxiety. Research shows that people victimized by workplace bullying had a four times higher risk of fibromyalgia.

Dr. Schubiner calls pain triggered by stress and emotion the Mind-Body Syndrome (MBS). "If you accept that your pain is triggered by learned nerve pathways formed during sustained negative emotional experiences and stress—by the MBS, and not by any physical illness or problem—you can then unlearn your pain, by learning to acknowledge and express your negative emotions, and by reducing stress."

Good news: The understanding of MBS and the techniques of ASA may help reduce pain in many of the 50 million Americans who suffer from chronic pain problems, including low back pain, sciatica, neck pain, whiplash, tendonitis, tension headache, migraine headaches and irritable bowel syndrome.

AFFIRM HEALTH, WRITE FREELY

Here are two techniques that can help you "unlearn" your pain, says Dr. Schubiner.

●**Affirm your essential health.** When pain or other symptoms occur, stop and take a deep breath. Then take a moment to remind yourself that there is nothing seriously wrong with your body. You are healthy, and the MBS symptoms will subside soon. Tell your mind that you realize that the symptoms are just a way of warning you about underlying feelings of fear, guilt, anger, anxiety, shame, inadequacy or other emotions. Tell your mind to stop producing the symptoms immediately. Do this with force and conviction, either out loud or silently. Take a few deep breaths, and move on with what you were doing.

For the greatest benefits: Repeat whatever positive phrases you choose every time you encounter any of your triggers, until your brain unlearns MBS pathways.

• **Write away your pain.** "Writing about stressful situations allows you to become healthier, develop perspective, and learn to let go of the emotional reactions that have imprisoned you," says Dr. Schubiner.

One such exercise is free-writing—writing faster than you normally would...writing whatever comes in your mind...allowing any thoughts and feelings to be expressed...not crossing out anything out...and not worrying about spelling, punctuation and grammar.

For ten minutes a day, free-write in response to the following sentences (use one sentence per day):

My feelings about me and _____ include:

My understandings about me and _____ include:

"The idea is to process your feelings," said Dr. Schubiner. "Expressing emotions is important, but it is also critical to understand them, gain perspective on them and begin to move past them.

"Therefore in this free-write, make sure to use phrases such as 'I see that...,' 'I realize...,' 'I hope that...,' 'I need to...,' 'I want to...,' 'I can...,' 'I will...,' 'I understand that...,' 'I appreciate...' 'I wonder if...,' 'I have learned...' and 'I have discovered...' "

Write whatever comes to your mind with a focus on understanding the topic/issue as best you can.

Once the ten minutes is up, complete the free-write by copying the following affirmation three times: Understanding these issues helps me feel better.

Resource: The same techniques used in the study are in the book *Unlearn Your Pain,* available at *www.unlearnyourpain.com,* where you can also enroll in Dr. Schubiner's Mind Body Program, read his blog and find other resources for overcoming MBS.

Sleeping Pill Helps Fibromyalgia and Chronic Fatigue

Relief for fibromyalgia and chronic fatigue symptoms may come from a prescription sleeping pill. Taken at bedtime, Xyrem (chemical name sodium oxybate) can help reduce the pain, fatigue, stiffness, disturbed sleep patterns and other symptoms associated with fibromyalgia and chronic fatigue syndrome (CFS). But Xyrem is not approved for this use—the FDA has approved it only for the treatment of narcolepsy (severe daytime sleepiness)—so insurers may not cover the cost unless it is needed for the FDA-approved purpose.

Less expensive alternative: The dietary supplement D-Ribose, available online and in health-food stores. It is a simple sugar found naturally in the body and may be even more effective than Xyrem.

Jacob Teitelbaum, MD, founder of the Practitioners Alliance Network. *Vitality101.com*

Good News for Fibromyalgia Sufferers!

In a recent study, 27 women with fibromyalgia received a low daily dose (4.5 mg) of *naltrexone* (Depade)—a drug normally used to treat narcotic addiction—for 12 weeks. They then took a placebo for four weeks. The drug reduced pain by an average of 48.5%, compared with 27.4% for the placebo.

Theory: Naltrexone may suppress functioning of hypersensitive immune cells, which can trigger fibromyalgia pain.

If you have fibromyalgia pain: Ask your doctor about an "off-label" prescription for naltrexone from a compounding pharmacy—the low dose used in the study isn't available at a regular pharmacy.

Jarred Younger, PhD, director of the Neuroinflammation, Pain and Fatigue Laboratory and associate professor in the psychology department at the College of Arts and Sciences at the University of Alabama at Birmingham.

Chronic Fatigue Helped by CoQ10

Belgian researchers have found that patients with myalgic encephalomyelitis/chronic fatigue syndrome, a range of illnesses characterized by extreme fatigue and muscle weakness, have very low blood levels of coenzyme Q10 (CoQ10), an antioxidant that helps cells function properly. CoQ10 may protect mitochondria, structures in cells that convert nutrients into energy. Patients with these disorders should supplement with CoQ10—other studies have shown it helps fatigue.

M. Maes, et al., "Coenzyme Q10 Deficiency in Myalgic Encephalomyelitis/Chronic Fatigue Syndrome (ME/CFS) Is Related to Fatigue, Autonomic and Neurocognitive Symptoms and Is Another Risk Factor Explaining the Early Mortality in ME/CFS Due to Cardiovascular Disorder," *Neuroendocrinology Letters.*

Fish Oil for Lupus

This chronic inflammatory disease can affect many body systems and organs.

Recent study: Lupus patients who took 3 grams of omega-3 fish oil supplements daily for 24 weeks showed significant improvement in lupus symptoms, such as fatigue, joint pain, skin rashes and mouth ulcers.

Cardiovascular benefits: There also was an improvement in blood vessel function and a reduction in cell-damaging molecules.

Best: Patients with lupus should ask their doctors about daily supplementation with omega-3 fish oils.

Stephen Wright, MD, group medical director/life-cycle leader at Genetech/Roche in South San Francisco, California, and lead investigator of a study on fish oils and lupus, presented at a meeting of the American College of Rheumatology.

Vitamin D Helps Lupus Patients

Researchers at Pitié-Salpêtrière Hospital, Paris, have found that very high doses of vitamin D (100,000 International Units) given once weekly for four weeks and then monthly for six months boosted the activity of helpful immune cells without causing unpleasant side effects. Lupus is an autoimmune disease that can affect joints and skin. Researchers caution patients with lupus against taking such high doses of vitamin D on their own. If you have lupus, speak to a holistic doctor about vitamin D therapy.

Mark A. Stengler, NMD, naturopathic medical doctor in private practice, Encinitas, California...adjunct associate clinical professor at the National College of Natural Medicine, Portland, Oregon...author of *The Natural Physician's Healing Therapies.*

The Painkiller Trap— Popular Drugs Can Make Your Pain Worse

Jane C. Ballantyne, MD, a professor in the department of anesthesiology and pain medicine at the University of Washington School of Medicine in Seattle, where she serves as director of the UW Pain Fellowship. She is coauthor of *Expert Decision Making on Opioid Treatment.*

If you have ever suffered from severe pain, you probably know that a strong pain pill can seem like the holy grail. In fact, with chronic pain affecting about one-third of Americans—or roughly 100 million people—it's perhaps no surprise that the most commonly prescribed opioid in the US is a painkiller, *hydrocodone* (Vicodin).

Frightening trend: Hydrocodone and the other prescription opioid painkillers (also known as narcotics) have now overtaken heroin and cocaine as the leading cause of fatal overdoses, according to the Centers for Disease Control and Prevention.

WHY THE SHIFT?

Until recently, prescription opioids were used to treat only acute (severe, short-lived) pain, such as pain after surgery or an injury or pain related to cancer.

Now: As doctors have stepped up their efforts to better control pain in all patients, opioids are more widely prescribed. These powerful medications are now being used to treat conditions such as low-back pain, chronic headaches and fibromyalgia.

What pain sufferers need to know...

DANGERS OF OPIOIDS

Each day, an estimated 4.3 million Americans take hydrocodone or other widely used opioids, such as *oxycodone* (OxyContin), *hydromorphone* (Dilaudid), codeine and morphine. For some patients, opioids are prescribed as an alternative to nonsteroidal anti-inflammatory drugs (NSAIDs), which are notorious for causing gastrointestinal bleeding and other side effects, including increased risk for heart attack and kidney disease.

Opioids work by mimicking natural pain-relieving chemicals in the body and attaching to receptors that block the transmission of pain messages to and within the brain. These drugs can be highly effective pain relievers, especially for arthritis patients who can't tolerate NSAIDs.

But opioids also have potentially serious side effects, especially when they're used long term (usually defined as more than 90 days). While the effectiveness of the medications often decreases over time (because the patient builds up a tolerance to the drug), the risk for side effects—including constipation, drowsiness or even addiction—increases due to the higher and more toxic doses used to overcome tolerance.

BEST NONDRUG ALTERNATIVES

If your doctor suggests taking an opioid for back pain, chronic headaches or migraines, or fibromyalgia, ask him/her about trying the following nondrug treatments first. Opioids should be considered only as a last resort.

• **Back pain.** For long-term low-back pain, exercises that strengthen the abdomen and back (or "core") muscles are the most effective treatment. If the pain is so severe that you can't exercise, over-the-counter painkillers sometimes can alleviate the pain enough to start an effective exercise regimen.

Bonus: Exercise can ease depression, which is common in back pain sufferers. Yoga may also be effective because it stretches the muscles and ligaments in addition to reducing mental stress.

Other possible options: If the approaches described above don't provide adequate relief, you may be a candidate for steroid injections into the spine or joints...a spinal fusion...or disk-replacement surgery. In general, these treatments have less risk for adverse effects than long-term use of opioids.

• **Chronic headaches or migraines.** With chronic headaches or migraines, opioids can worsen pain by causing "rebound" headaches that occur when the drug is overused. Try lifestyle changes, such as daily meditation, and the sparing use of mild painkillers, such as NSAIDs. Supplements, including magnesium and feverfew, also have been shown to relieve headache pain.

• **Fibromyalgia.** With this condition, which has no known cure, opioids have been found to intensify existing pain.

Much better: A review of 46 studies has found aerobic exercise, such as brisk walking or pool aerobics (done two to three times a week for an hour), may reduce system-wide inflammation, making it an effective treatment for fibromyalgia.

If you're in too much pain to do aerobic exercise, a mild painkiller or a nondrug approach, such as massage, may allow you to start.

Cognitive behavioral therapy is another good choice. With this treatment, a therapist can help you reframe negative thoughts that may be fueling fibromyalgia pain.

Additional nondrug approaches that may help all of these conditions: Acupuncture, relaxation exercises and heating pads.

4

De-Stress and Energize Your Life

Your "Stress Type" Holds the Key to Stress Relief

We all know that chronic stress is linked to many health problems, from heart disease to cancer to autoimmune disorders to depression. But simply telling ourselves to "de-stress" is distressingly ineffective...and since we don't all experience stress the same way, what works for one woman may do nothing for another.

What does help: A personalized approach based on an individual's "stress type," Stephanie McClellan, MD, coauthor of *So Stressed: The Ultimate Stress-Relief Plan for Women*, has identified four basic stress types...the biochemical imbalances behind each...and specific lifestyle strategies that bring relief. *Two main factors combine to determine your stress* type...

• **Your levels of the stress hormone cortisol.** The "hyper" stress types have too much cortisol, while "hypo" stress types have too little. Though you may think of cortisol as

"bad," it is essential for normal brain and body function—so too much or too little can affect energy level, emotions and immune function, Dr. McClellan explained.

• **Which part of your nervous system is dominant.** Dr. McClellan refers to people in whom the sympathetic nervous system (which controls the fight-or-flight response) is constantly aroused as "S" stress types. In contrast, with the "P" stress types, the parasympathetic nervous system (which induces the rest-and-restore function) overshoots its target, depleting energy and norepinephrine, a brain chemical linked to arousal, attention, memory and mood.

Here's how to tell which stress type you are and what to do to feel and function better.

Stephanie McClellan, MD, is a gynecologist in private practice and former chairman of the department of obstetrics and gynecology and cofounder of the Women's Health Pavilion at Hoag Memorial Hospital Presbyterian in Newport Beach, California. She is the coauthor, with Beth Hamilton, MD, of *So Stressed: The Ultimate Stress-Relief Plan for Women*.

You are a "Hyper S" woman in overdrive if you…

• **Are always on the go,** even when exhausted…and treat nearly every task as an emergency.

• **Feel anxious,** irritable and fidgety.

• **Are prone to headaches,** sinus infections, heart palpitations, acne and/or insomnia.

What's going on: This stress type is characterized by high cortisol levels and an overactive sympathetic nervous system.

De-stress dietary tactic: To boost levels of the calming neurotransmitter serotonin, eat foods that contain the amino acids tryptophan (beef, cheese, chicken, eggs, fish, soybeans, turkey, yogurt) and tyrosine (avocados, bananas, carrots, game meats, nuts). Avoid coffee—instead, have green tea or white tea, which has far less caffeine and also provides L-theanine, an amino acid that promotes a relaxed, yet alert, mental state.

Best exercise strategy: To release pent-up energy, work out vigorously for at least 30 minutes five or more times a week. Exercise in the morning, Dr. McClellan suggested, when your body is naturally producing more cortisol for the energy you need to get through the day. Anything that gets your heart pumping will do—brisk walking, cycling, using an elliptical machine.

Targeted relaxation techniques: The goal is to quiet your overstimulated mind and relax tense muscles. For at least five minutes three times daily, try mindfulness meditation, paying attention moment by moment to whatever crosses your mind, without judgment or analysis…or progressive muscle relaxation, tensing and then relaxing muscles, body part by body part.

You are a "Hyper P" dash-and-crasher if you…

• **Are a high achiever,** pushing yourself relentlessly…then, after the stressful situation passes, you "crash"—experiencing extreme exhaustion that leaves you temporarily unable to function.

• **Feel overemotional,** unfocused and withdrawn when burned out.

• **Are prone to colds,** flu and/or blurry vision…and often get sick on vacations.

What's going on: High cortisol and a dominant parasympathetic nervous system define this stress type. As your nervous system swings from high gear to crashing, norepinephrine is depleted and immune function is compromised.

De-stress dietary tactic: To build up your weakened immune system, eat lots of antioxidant-packed fruits and vegetables and foods rich in zinc (cashews, cheese, chicken liver, shellfish). To restore energy, stabilize blood sugar levels by breakfasting on protein-rich foods (eggs, yogurt) and eating small meals and snacks throughout the day.

Best exercise strategy: When you feel near collapse, refrain from strenuous exercise for a few days—just take leisurely walks or do gentle yoga poses. Once you feel stronger, follow the Hyper S woman's exercise plan mentioned earlier.

Targeted relaxation techniques: Pamper yourself when drained by taking a long bath or getting a massage or manicure…and/or try prayer to lift your spirits, Dr. McClelland suggested.

You are a fried-and-frazzled "Hypo S" type if you…

• **Appear outwardly calm but dread conflict or pressure.**

• **Are anxious and fearful when stressed…** and often feel like you don't get enough sleep.

• **May have aches and pains,** allergies, thyroid problems, lupus and/or arthritis.

What's going on: The low cortisol associated with this stress type leads to an overactive immune system…while the overly excitable sympathetic nervous system creates extreme sensitivity to stress.

De-stress dietary tactic: Make lunch your main meal—this helps boost cortisol levels— and focus on lean protein and complex carbohydrates (whole grains, legumes). To calm your immune system, eat foods rich in inflammation-fighting omega-3 fatty acids (fish, olive oil, walnuts). Have a bit of dark chocolate—it can encourage production of pain-relieving endorphins, Dr. McClellan said.

Best exercise strategy: Lack of energy makes exercising tough, but aim for 30 minutes three times a week—it will help reduce pains, make your brain less stress-sensitive and increase endorphins and mood-elevating serotonin. Try rhythmic, low-impact activities—ballroom dancing, swimming, cycling or even a walk outside, which are soothing yet relieve sluggishness.

Targeted relaxation techniques: The focus is on reducing pain and raising energy. Try aromatherapy…slow deep breathing…and reflexology, in which pressure is applied to certain points on the feet to unblock energy flow.

You are a detached and shut-down "Hypo P" type if you…

• **Are passive in the face of adversity…**and have trouble expressing emotions.

• **Feel unstimulated and detached,** like a spectator in your own life.

• **Are chronically exhausted…**often feel dizzy, faint or achy…and/or suffer from gastrointestinal upsets.

What's going on: This is the rarest stress type, a mix of low cortisol, low norepinephrine and a chronically understimulated stress response.

De-stress dietary tactic: Eat easy-to-digest foods—high-fiber fruits and whole grains, cooked vegetables (rather than raw), dairy foods made with sheep's milk (instead of cow's milk). Talk to your doctor about supplementing with vitamin A and vitamin E because you may not be absorbing enough of these from your food.

Best exercise strategy: You're so tired that it's hard to work out, so start with a daily five-minute walk outside to get the mood-boosting benefit of sunshine…a 20-minute stretch…or lifting two-pound weights while you watch TV. Exercise (preferably in natural sunlight) at the same time each day to regulate cortisol production. As energy increases, gradually ramp up your workout.

Targeted relaxation techniques: Restoration is your priority. Keep a journal to explore

bottled-up emotions…try Shiatsu massage, which focuses on acupressure points and unblocks energy meridians. If you feel depressed, work with a mental health professional to rediscover vitality and joy.

An Ancient Secret That Makes Driving Stress-Free

Catherine Hilker is a certified feng shui consultant based in the Detroit area and the Red Ribbon Professional Consultant of the International Feng Shui Guild. *CatherineBilker.com*

Whether you love to drive or despise it, there's no denying that driving can be stressful at times. Believe it or not, there are ancient principles that can transform your car's interior into an environment that is relaxing and enjoyable—and safe. The secret lies in *feng shui,* the Chinese art of positioning objects to create harmonious, peaceful surroundings.

Feng shui is commonly thought of as applying to the arrangement of furniture and other items in a home or office, but there's no reason you can't extend the concepts to your car, too. And there's no need to buy a new vehicle—you can get the stress-easing benefits of feng shui in your current car, yet spend little or nothing, by making some simple changes.

To discuss the specifics, we spoke with Catherine Hilker, a certified feng shui consultant and professional consultant of the International Feng Shui Guild. She explained that feng shui involves the concept of yin and yang, the two complementary forces that make up all aspects of the universe. For instance, yin is earth, femaleness, darkness and passivity… yang is heaven, maleness, light and activity. Ideally, yin and yang are in harmony.

Ours tends to be a yang culture, however, Hilker noted. Many Americans are impatient, prone to cram schedules too full and drive too fast. Not only is this an extreme and out-of-balance expression of yang, but such behaviors can be very dangerous while driving. And even if you are not this way yourself, other drivers often are—so you're still likely to be stressed on the road.

The way to adjust extreme yang in a car is to bring in yin elements, said Hilker. Here's how...

• **Clear away clutter.** "A disarrayed, dirty or cluttered environment produces si chi, or decaying energy, which depletes the body's own chi, or vital energy, creating pressure or tension," Hilker explained. So get rid of the empty water bottles, food wrappers, newspapers and other junk...organize a kit to neatly hold maps, flashlights, pens and other items...vacuum carpets and seats...keep windows clean and unobstructed.

• **Add touches of the right color to your car's interior environment.** Across the seat, spread a blanket or scarf of appropriate yin colors.

Examples: Black or very dark colors help you slow down...earth tones keep you feeling grounded and stable...blue is soothing and calming. Avoid yang colors, such as red and very bright hues.

• **Carry a meaningful icon or symbol.** You might choose an object that represents safety, tranquility, courtesy, groundedness or good fortune—for instance, a small medal or statue of St. Christopher (patron saint of travelers)...an object of nature, such as a stone, crystal or animal figurine...or a favorite good luck charm. If you find a spot where your icon can be seen without being distracting or looking like clutter, put it there...otherwise, tuck it away in the glove box and take it out when you need to destress.

• **Fill your ears with soothing sounds.** "When you are in a car, avoid news reports and harsh music—these create a negative vibe in a vehicle, and negativity attracts more negativity," Hilker said.

Better: Listen to chi-enhancing soft music or nature sounds while you drive.

• **Be safe.** Keep your car in top working condition...never text while driving...don't get sucked into potentially upsetting phone calls or conversations with passengers when

you're behind the wheel. After all, feeling safe in your surroundings is an essential aspect of feng shui.

10-Minute Ritual for All-Day Energy

Nancy Lonsdorf, MD, ABIHM (board certified by the American Board of Integrative Holistic Medicine), is an Ayurvedic doctor specializing in healthy longevity and women's issues. She is an associate clinical professor at Maharishi University of Management in Fairfield, Iowa, author of *The Ageless Woman: Natural Health and Beauty After Forty with Maharishi Ayurveda* and a coauthor of *A Woman's Best Medicine: Health, Happiness, and Long Life through Maharishi Ayurveda.* DrLonsdorf.com/

Do you often feel sluggish, fatigued, foggy-brained or blue? There's a potential solution that is simple, takes as little as 10 minutes per day and costs absolutely nothing, according to Nancy Lonsdorf, MD, who practices Ayurveda, a system of natural medicine based on the premise that nature knows best.

The secret: Take a walk outdoors in the fresh air, for at least 10 minutes, within an hour or two of dawn.

"The rising sun and morning air are invigorating because they are filled with what Ayurveda calls prana, or life force. This gives you energy and clears out any morning brain fog. It has a revitalizing effect on the emotions, too, creating a positive mood for the whole day. A dawn walk also enhances *ojas*, a subtle essence of the physical body that helps keep you fully immune and strengthened against disease," said Dr. Lonsdorf. From the perspective of Western medicine, she added, an early morning walk gets your circulation and metabolism going after you have been asleep all night and also is good for digestion.

The practice may even have beauty benefits, too. "After taking one of my seminars, a kindergarten teacher went for a walk early the next morning. When she got to school, a student said, 'You look so pretty today!' She hadn't done anything different with her makeup, hair or clothes—the only change was that sunrise walk," Dr. Lonsdorf said.

For best effect: Get up by 6 am (called *vata* time in the Ayurvedic tradition). Then walk toward the rising sun, letting its light fall on your face. And don't worry about the weather—no matter whether it's hot or cold, sunny or rainy or snowing outside, your dawn walk will be richly rewarding.

Feel Like You've Got More Hours in Your Day

Melanie Rudd, PhD, is a consumer psychologist, assistant professor of marketing and entrepreneurship, University of Houston, C.T. Bauer College of Business in Texas and lead author of an article on awe and time perception published in *Psychological Science*.

Think back to a moment when you felt utterly awestruck by the splendor of a sunset, the majesty of a symphony or the miracle of a newborn baby. Remember how it seemed as though time stood still while your mind and soul expanded to absorb the immensity of the experience?

Well, when you tap into that type of feeling, you can find relief from a scourge of modern existence—the sense of being constantly starved for time. And in so doing, you may boost your satisfaction with life and even improve your health!

This fascinating finding comes from a new study that examined the power of awe, the emotion that arises when we encounter something so strikingly vast that it alters our understanding of the world. (Yes, scientists study awe—you gotta love it!) *The study included three experiments with three different sets of participants…*

●**Experiment #1.** Volunteers were randomly assigned to watch a one-minute video designed to elicit either awe or happiness. (Happiness was chosen as the basis of comparison because it also is a positive emotion but does not share awe's mind-altering immensity.) The awe-inspiring video showed waterfalls, whales and astronauts in space…the happiness-inspiring video showed a parade of joyful people.

When surveyed afterward: Compared with participants who felt happy, those who felt awed were more likely to agree with statements such as, "I have lots of time in which I can get things done"—showing that they perceived time as more plentiful.

●**Experiment #2.** One group of participants wrote about an occasion when they experienced awe…a second group wrote about an occasion when they felt happy. Then they answered questionnaires to determine their levels of impatience and their willingness to donate time to help other people.

Results: Members of the awe group were significantly less impatient and more willing to spend time helping others—indicating that they felt as though they had time to spare.

●**Experiment #3.** Volunteers read a story about climbing the Eiffel Tower and admiring Paris from on high (to inspire awe)…or they read about climbing an unnamed tower and seeing a plain landscape (a neutral experience). Afterward, they made hypothetical choices between material goods or enjoyable experiences—for instance, a wristwatch versus tickets to a Broadway show—and answered questions about how satisfied they felt with life at that moment.

Findings: The awe group favored experiences (which take time but generally deliver more long-lasting satisfaction than material goods)…and reported greater life satisfaction overall.

What it all means: Researchers noted that people who feel rushed tend to eat less healthfully…often forgo leisure activities and community service…and are at increased risk for high blood pressure, headaches, stomach pain, poor sleep and depression.

Antidote for the time famine: By actively pursuing and/or consciously recalling awe-inspiring experiences, we can seemingly slow the rush of time and find more joy and meaning in our lives. So why not take a few moments to read an epic poem or admire a star-spangled sky…and let yourself be filled with wonder.

Laugh Your Way to Better Health

Katherine Puckett, PhD, is the chief, division of mind-body medicine at the Cancer Treatment Centers of America facility at Midwestern Regional Medical Center in Zion, Illinois. She is a licensed clinical social worker and certified laughter leader.

Have you ever laughed and then said, "Thanks, I needed that"? You were so right—because the very act of laughing promotes good health in numerous ways. And in fact, you can maximize these health benefits for yourself by doing fun and simple "laughter exercises."

Want evidence of how laughter helps? Consider a recent study at Loma Linda University, which involved diabetic patients who had high cholesterol and high blood pressure. One group of participants received standard pharmaceutical treatment for these conditions...a second group received the same medications but also were instructed to "view self-selected humor" (for instance, watch sitcoms or videos that they considered funny) for 30 minutes daily.

After one year: In the laughter group, HDL (good) cholesterol increased by 26% and blood levels of C reactive protein (a marker of inflammation) decreased by 66%, on average... in the other group, HDL increased by just 3% and C-reactive protein declined by just 26%, on average.

Additional research from Loma Linda University suggests that laughter also can boost immunity...relax tense muscles...reduce levels of stress hormones...and raise levels of mood-elevating hormones called endorphins (the same hormones released during orgasm!).

It is easy to bring more laughter to your life. "The average adult laughs 17 times daily. Keep track for a few days—and if you're not laughing at least that often, make a conscious effort to increase your opportunities to laugh," suggested Katherine Puckett, PhD, chief of mind-body medicine at the Cancer Treatment Centers of America facility in Zion, Illinois, who has extensive experience applying therapeutic laughter. "Since we laugh most frequently during social interactions with others, spend time with people who enjoy laughing and being playful. Also try watching children and pets playing...enjoying funny videos... deliberately smiling more often (it's contagious!)...and observing the world through a 'comic lens' as you look for humor around you even in difficult situations."

Another option is to consciously do laughter exercises with friends, family or coworkers. If you feel self-conscious at first, remind yourselves that you're laughing with each other, not at each other, and that your intention is to have good-natured fun. "At first, the laughter is simulated—but in short order, it becomes real," Dr. Puckett said. *As often as you like, try...*

● **Laughter chant.** As you clap in rhythm, repeatedly say, "Ho-ho ha-ha-ha, ho-ho ha-ha-ha."

● **Roller coaster.** Lift your arms, sway, jiggle and scream as if you were on a coaster. (This is easiest while seated.)

● **Snowball fight.** Lean over and scoop up some imaginary snow, pack it into a snowball and throw it at another person. Everyone naturally laughs while throwing or being "hit." Try putting some pretend snow down someone's back, which may make you both laugh even harder.

● **Sing with laughter.** Even if no one is having a birthday, sing Happy Birthday to You to each other, substituting "hee hee" or "ha ha" or "ho ho" for each word. You can swap this laughter vocabulary for the words in many songs—and before you even finish singing, you'll be feeling happier and more energized.

How to Restore Your Energy Without Sleeping

Matthew Edlund, MD, sleep, biological clocks, performance and rest expert, and author of *The Power of Rest: Why Sleep Alone Is Not Enough.* He is director of the Center for Circadian Medicine, Sarasota, Florida.

Matthew Edlund, MD, author of the book *The Power of Rest: Why Sleep Alone Is Not Enough,* is a proponent of what he calls "powerful resting," which involves a lot more than snoozing, reading or watching TV. "Rest doesn't mean just immobility," he explains. "It is anything we do with the intention of regenerating the body." There are other ways of resting, he says, that can help you increase productivity and improve your mood, health and pleasure—and even help you maintain a healthy weight.

In Dr. Edlund's view, lying around on the couch or sleeping are classic examples of passive rest—which has value, of course. However, Dr. Edlund's primary focus is something else—the pursuit of active rest. This includes activities and exercises that he describes as "restorative in that they rebuild and rewire body and mind…let you retune and reset…and consciously direct your body and brain to be more capable of doing whatever you want to do."

A common mistake people make is to consider active rest as little more than engaging in "fun activities," such as the things we all tend to do on vacations. But that view is incomplete, he says. In fact, active rest is not just fun—it contributes to longevity and health by creating a better mood and balance in your life as well as reducing stress. In Dr. Edlund's mind, that is why it should be a regular part of our lives.

EXERCISES FOR ACTIVE REST

Dr. Edlund has identified four life areas that provide opportunities for active rest and offered a specific exercise to experience and enhance each of them…

•**Physical rest.** Sleep is just one part of physical rest, Dr. Edlund points out. He suggests that we all can benefit from performing simple physiological tasks while we are awake to bring a calm, relaxed state and mental alertness—without taking a nap.

Suggested activity: "Paradoxical Relaxation." Close your eyes and feel the motion of your eyeballs, which will automatically continue to move under your closed lids. Target any area of your body where you can feel muscle tension—if you can't think of one, try your left eye (or the right one if you are left-handed, since it is easier to focus on the body part that you don't automatically use). Keep your mental focus there, and experience the intensity of

tension as the muscle moves—without trying to modify or change it in any way. Do this for several minutes, then shift your focus to another area of tension in a different body part, such as your neck, shoulder or hand, where you will repeat the same activity.

Benefit: The paradoxical aspect of this exercise is that paying attention to one specific area of tension, in this case your eye, relaxes muscles throughout the entire body. This can be a good trick to help you get to sleep as well.

•**Mental rest.** Actively resting your mind quickly produces relaxation and focus that can bring greater awareness, concentration and achievement.

Suggested activity: "Walking to Music." Find a place where you have enough space to walk around comfortably for about one minute, such as a long hallway, a parking lot or, better yet, a park. But before walking, use a portable music player or just your imagination to "listen to" one fast tune and a slow one for about 30 seconds as you stand without moving. Then replay (on your device or in your head) the fast song and walk with its rhythm, getting your whole body into the beat. After you really start to feel it in your body (for most people, that's about 20 seconds), switch to the slow song for the same period of time and adjust your gait accordingly. Notice how different your muscles feel and how each tune affects your mood. If you're feeling good, you can continue this exercise longer and feel even more enlivened.

Benefit: Walking to music takes you away from your current thoughts and worries while also focusing your brain and engaging your muscles simultaneously. This in turn produces a quick boost of energy and activates the pleasure center of the brain (like dancing does). It will improve your mood!

•**Social rest.** The power of social rest comes from connecting with others, thus creating feelings of belonging and togetherness, both of which promote good health.

Suggested activity: Walk to lunch with a colleague, friend or neighbor. To do this, consider who in your life you would like to know better and spend more time with—say a co-worker who is really in the know about your workplace, a neighbor who is full of good cheer, a friend who has long been special to you. Every few weeks, invite one of them to lunch. Here is the catch—you are to choose a place for lunch that takes about 10 minutes to walk to. As you walk to and from the restaurant with your companion, let him or her do most of the chatting initially while you pay close attention not only to the words but also to his or her carriage and posture, facial expressions and emotions.

Benefit: Focusing on someone else can take you deeper into the dynamics and flow of your relationships and at the same time remove you from a focus on your own life, producing a relaxing and enriching break.

●**Spiritual rest.** This type of rest connects you to larger and greater aspects of life (such as a higher power) while also promoting a sense of internal balance.

Suggested activity: "Moving through Time and Space." This is a journey of the imagination that will take three to five minutes. As you sit at your table or desk, close your eyes and picture life as it was in that specific location one year ago…10 years ago…100 years…1,000 years…and finally reaching all the way back to prehistoric times and then beyond, to the time before everything began. Stay in each time period for a few seconds before reversing the pattern and, just as quickly, moving forward. Then take another mental "trip," but this time, focus on internal space, beginning by picturing your heart…then zooming in to the left side of it and the valves there…then the arteries…the blood vessel branches…the cells…the molecules…and, finally, the atoms. Once again, reverse the pattern—now quickly imagining your internal structure from the tiniest elements and zooming out to your heart in the present.

Benefit: This provides perspective and a sense of awe about the vastness of the universe as you take yourself backward and then hurtle forward through time and space.

Each of these activities—and others that Dr. Edlund describes in his book—takes only a few minutes to accomplish. They are easy to fit into your day whenever you feel the need to "power up," as he puts it. You can catch your breath by calming down, bringing the focus back to who you are—all truly regenerative and restorative, just as he says.

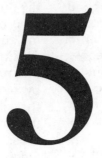

5

Fix the Aches and Pains of Daily Life

Hands-On Help for Tension Headaches

An argument with your spouse, an impossible deadline at work, a traffic jam that makes you miss a long-awaited appointment—these are the types of everyday stresses that can lead to tension headaches. Nearly everyone gets them at one time or another. And since women are more prone to this problem than men, you're probably familiar with the symptoms—viselike pain or dull pressure that starts in the forehead or temple area and spreads over the entire head...plus tightness in the neck, shoulders and/or jaw. Symptoms typically last about half an hour, though they can persist for days.

Why not just pop a pill to get rid of the pain? Because doing so can actually make the problem worse, given that people who take over-the-counter or prescription pain medication more than three days a week on a regular basis may develop rebound headaches. Pain

relievers also have potentially serious side effects, including increased risk for gastrointestinal bleeding, blood pressure problems, and kidney or liver damage.

Safer, speedy solutions: Hands-on techniques you can do yourself often relieve tension headaches within minutes, according to neurologist Trupti Gokani, MD, founder of the Zira Mind and Body Center in Glenview, Illinois.

You can try the methods below in any order. Unless otherwise indicated, continue with any given technique for about three minutes. Dr. Gokani noted that patients often try a technique for less than a minute and then give up—but it takes time to modify the stress response that the body naturally enters into when pain is perceived. It also is important to relax and breathe while doing the techniques, she added...simple oxygenation helps quiet

---

Trupti Gokani, MD, is a board-certified neurologist and founder of the Zira Mind and Body Center in Glenview, Illinois. Her special interests include alternative approaches to headache management and women's issues. *ZiraMindAndBody.com*

down the brain and relieve pain. If one technique does not help, try another. With a bit of experimentation, you'll soon discover what works best for you.

●**Acupressure.** This soothes symptoms by easing muscle tension and/or triggering the release of pain-relieving endorphins. Pressure points to try…

●The base of the skull. With hands interlaced at the back of your head, place your thumbs at the base of the skull where you feel the indentations on both sides of the neck muscle. Press with your thumbs—first gently, then with increasing pressure—breathing deeply and slowly tilting your head back.

●The loose, webby skin between your thumb and index finger, about an inch from the edge. Using your right thumb and index finger, tightly squeeze this spot on the left hand (you may find it tender), massaging the area in small circles…then switch hands.

●Above each eye, just beneath the center of each eyebrow. Use your thumbs to gently probe the area, looking for a small groove in the skull at the top of each eye socket—you'll find a nerve that is very sensitive to pressure. Once you locate the right spot, carefully apply pressure for just five to 10 seconds—it will hurt, but the discomfort stimulates the pituitary gland to release endorphins.

●**Warm compress.** Applied directly, heat helps relax muscles and therefore alleviates tension headache pain. Dr. Gokani suggested placing a warm, wet cloth or a microwavable heat pack on your forehead…if desired, place a second warm compress at the back of your neck.

●**Yoga poses.** If you are an experienced yogini, check out the advanced headache-relieving poses at *www.YogaJournal.com. Otherwise, place a mat or blanket on the floor and try these simple options…*

●Child's pose. This promotes all-over relaxation and is especially effective at alleviating facial tension. Kneel with your knees hip-width apart and big toes touching…sit back on your heels…lean forward, resting your torso between your thighs…gently rest your forehead on the ground…rest your arms alongside your shins,

palms up. Illustration: *www.YogaJournal.com/ poses/475.*

●Cat and cow stretch. These poses help release neck and back tension. Start on hands and knees, with your wrists directly below your shoulders and your knees directly below your hips. Exhaling, round your spine toward the ceiling, releasing your head toward the floor (cat pose)…then, as you inhale, allow your belly to drop toward the floor as you arch your back and lift your head to look straight forward (cow pose). Continue slowly and smoothly alternating between these two poses, holding each pose for a count of 10. Illustrations: *www.YogaJournal. com/poses/2468* and *www.YogaJournal.com/ poses/2467.*

Final note: If you experience severe, frequent or unremitting headaches, it is important to see your physician to check for possible underlying causes, Dr. Gokani said. However, for many people, one or more of the strategies above will be sufficient to provide speedy relief from tension headache pain.

What to Take for a Tension Headache— No Drugs Needed

Trupti Gokani, MD, is a board-certified neurologist and founder of the Zira Mind and Body Center in Glenview, Illinois. Her special interests include alternative approaches to headache management and women's issues. *ZiraMindAndBody.com*

Its trivial-sounding name seems to imply that the problem is "just stress"…but the viselike pain of a tension headache can make you truly miserable and significantly disrupt your day. Popping a painkiller is not a great solution because such drugs can have nasty side effects, including increased risk for gastrointestinal bleeding, blood pressure problems and liver or kidney damage.

So what can you take when a tension headache grabs hold? Integrative neurologist Trupti Gokani, MD, founder of the Zira Mind and Body Center in Glenview, suggested trying any or all of the following options. Products are available at health-food stores and/or online. *Consider taking…*

•**A few bites of food or a big drink of water.** If hunger or dehydration is triggering your headache, the pain may disappear once you assuage your body's basic needs. Just about any healthful food will do…but stay away from known headache triggers such as processed meats, aged cheeses, red wine and anything with monosodium glutamate, Dr. Gokani said.

•**Butterbur supplements.** Though various supplements may prevent headaches when taken regularly (and we'll discuss these options another day), Dr. Gokani said that butterbur works best to help halt a headache you already have. This anti-inflammatory herb should be taken as soon as you feel the pain coming on. Try the brand Petadolex (*www.Pet adolex.com*), which contains a purified form of butterbur free from liver-damaging pyrrolizidine alkaloids. Or consider Zira Nourished Mind by PureBalance, a product Dr. Gokani helped develop, which contains Petadolex and other headache-relieving ingredients (available at *www.ziramindandbody.com/products*).

Caution: Do not use butterbur if you are pregnant or have liver disease.

•**Some whiffs of an aromatherapy remedy.** Finding the right scent may require some experimentation, Dr. Gokani said, because an aroma that soothes pain for one person can irritate another.

Options to try: Essential oil of lavender…basil…or clary sage.

To use: Sprinkle three drops of the desired essential oil onto a tissue or handkerchief and take a sniff every few minutes…or sprinkle three drops onto a hot or cold compress and apply to your forehead until the pain lets up.

•**A moment to ask yourself why you have this headache.** A tension headache usually has an underlying trigger, Dr. Gokani noted.

Consider: Do you need a break from your computer screen? Are you working in a poorly lit room? Might a short walk or a chat with a friend help relieve whatever stress you're under? Once you identify the root problem and take action to rectify it, your pain should ease up.

Extreme Migraine Makeover

Among migraine patients who had forehead surgery to remove muscles at headache trigger sites, 57% reported permanent elimination of migraines (compared with 4% of a control group who had sham surgery)…and 84% had at least a 50% reduction in symptoms. Side effects included temporary facial numbness and, rarely, very slight (and fixable) hollowing of the temples.

Bonus: The operation, similar to a forehead lift, reduced forehead wrinkles.

Good news: This surgery, which is now available, offers hope for migraine patients who want to avoid or do not respond to medication. Many insurance companies cover at least a portion of the cost.

Bahman Guyuron, MD, emeritus professor, department of plastic surgery, Case Western Reserve University School of Medicine in Cleveland and author of seven studies on surgical treatment for migraine.

No More Migraines

Mark A. Stengler, NMD, is a naturopathic medical doctor, author of *The Natural Physician's Healing Therapies*, founder and medical director of the Stengler Center for Integrative Medicine in Encinitas, California, and adjunct associate clinical professor at the National College of Natural Medicine in Portland, Oregon. *MarkStengler.com*

Using the word headache to describe a migraine is like referring to the space shuttle as an airplane. Technically, migraines are headaches, of course—but the suffering they cause far exceeds that of most other types. An estimated 30 million Americans, most of them between ages 15 and 55, get migraines. Women sufferers outnumber men three to one, and while the onset of menopause sometimes brings relief, it doesn't always. Fewer than half of migraine sufferers are properly diagnosed—instead, many are incorrectly told that their headaches stem from sinus problems or tension. Because treatments for other types of headaches do not alleviate migraines, millions of people suffer needlessly.

Standard treatment for migraines includes prescription drugs, such as *sumatriptan* (Imitrex), *zolmitriptan* (Zomig) and *rizatriptan* (Maxalt). These are intended to prevent, halt or ease migraines—but they do not work for everyone. Potential side effects include nausea, dizziness, diarrhea and sweating...and in rare cases, an increased risk for heart attack and stroke, perhaps due to blood vessel damage. When the drugs are discontinued, patients may get rebound headaches.

Good news: It is possible to reduce the frequency of migraines or prevent them by using natural, nutritional, drug-free substances.

GETTING THE RIGHT DIAGNOSIS

Migraines occur when arteries in the brain dilate abnormally and nerves that coil around the arteries are stretched. In response, the nerves release chemicals that cause painful inflammation and further enlargement of arteries, magnifying pain even more.

Migraine symptoms are distinct from those of other types of headaches. If you experience two or more of the following symptoms, you probably are dealing with migraines. *Migraine pain may*...

• **Occur on one side of the head.**
• **Last from four hours to as long as 72 hours.**
• **Pulsate or throb.**
• **Be triggered by certain foods or situations.**
• **Worsen during exertion, such as when climbing stairs.**
• **Be accompanied by nausea or vomiting.**
• **Be exacerbated by sound.**
• **Be accompanied by oversensitivity to light.**

About 20% of migraine sufferers experience aura, a visual disturbance that typically comes on 20 to 60 minutes before the onset of pain. Aura may be perceived as flashing lights, blind spots or wavy lines in the field of vision. It may be accompanied by facial tingling, muscle weakness and/or speech difficulties, such as slurring words or having trouble finding words. Aura occurs when certain nerve cells in the brain become temporarily hyperactive, triggering visual disturbances and tingling sensations...while in other nerve cells, activity is depressed, temporarily impairing vision, speech and muscle strength.

Another clue: Up to 80% of migraine sufferers have a family history of the condition—so if a close relative has migraines, you are more likely to get them, too.

If you suspect migraines, see a headache specialist or neurologist. He/she should take a detailed history that includes your migraine symptoms...pattern of attacks...other types of headaches you have...family history of headaches...and all of your medications, because those that affect circulation (such as hypertension drugs and birth control pills) can contribute to migraines. Hormone testing may be appropriate, as deficiencies of estrogen and/or progesterone (in women) or of thyroid hormone can lead to migraines. All of this information is vital, because no tests can definitively confirm a migraine diagnosis.

NATURAL WAYS TO PREVENT MIGRAINES

Numerous studies confirm the benefits of the vitamin-like coenzyme Q10 (CoQ10)...riboflavin (vitamin B-2)...and the mineral magnesium. Taking just one of these three natural substances can decrease migraine severity and/or frequency by about half. In my experience, when patients regularly take all three, overall improvement can exceed 75%.

Theory: An abnormal lag in brain cells' energy production triggers the blood vessel dilation that leads to a migraine. These three nutrients support the mitochondria—structures in cells that convert oxygen and nutrients into chemical energy to power the cells' metabolic activities—helping them to work more effectively and thereby preventing migraines.

Daily prevention strategy: I suggest using all three of these substances if you get migraines once or more per month. Take them for four months. If you notice improvement, continue indefinitely. Dosages and guidelines for people age 12 and up...

•**CoQ10 at 100 mg three times daily.** Occasional side effects, such as mild heartburn or nausea, can be avoided by taking CoQ10 with meals.

•**Riboflavin at 400 mg once daily.** B vitamins work best when in balance with one another, so take an additional B complex or multivitamin.

•**Magnesium at 200 mg twice daily (reduce dosage if you develop diarrhea).** Least likely to cause loose stool is the magnesium glycinate form.

These supplements are sold in health-food stores, are nontoxic, rarely have side effects and generally are safe. *Evidence that they work...*

•**CoQ10.** In a study published in the journal *Cephalalgia*, 31 migraine patients took 150 mg of CoQ10 daily. After three months, the number of migraine attacks fell, on average, from 4.85 to 2.81 per month...and duration of pain (measured in "migraine days") was significantly reduced. In another study, Swiss and Belgian researchers gave 42 patients a placebo or CoQ10 at 100 mg three times daily for three months. Migraine frequency fell by at least half in 47% of patients taking CoQ10, compared with 14% of the placebo group. CoQ10 users also had less nausea.

•**Riboflavin.** In a Belgian study, 55 migraine patients took either a placebo or 400 mg of riboflavin daily. Frequency and duration of migraines decreased by at least half in 59% of riboflavin users, compared with 15% of placebo users. Research suggests that combining riboflavin with beta-blockers (cardiovascular drugs sometimes prescribed for migraines) may be more effective at preventing migraines than either therapy used alone.

•**Magnesium.** Up to half of patients have a deficiency of magnesium during a migraine, as shown by testing of blood drawn during attacks. Oral magnesium supplementation may reduce the frequency and duration of migraines.

Possible reason: Upon exposure to a migraine trigger, excess calcium flows into brain cells, causing a sudden constriction of blood vessels...and magnesium supplementation combats this by normalizing the balance of minerals in the brain. In addition, intravenous (IV) magnesium can give fast relief from acute migraine symptoms. Although conventional doctors generally do not offer this therapy, some holistic practitioners do.

MIGRAINE TRIGGERS

In susceptible individuals, certain foods and/or situations can bring on a migraine. To identify your triggers, keep a diary for four weeks, noting when your migraines occur and looking for patterns.

Common food culprits...

•**Alcohol, especially red wine and beer**
•**Caffeine**
•**Chocolate**
•**Cheese,** especially aged (Parmesan, Asiago)
•**Fermented foods** (miso, sauerkraut)
•**Monosodium glutamate** (a flavoring)
•**Nitrates** (a type of preservative)
•**Pickled foods** (dill pickles, olives, capers)
•**Shellfish**
•**Wheat**

SITUATIONAL TRIGGERS

•**Changes in weather, altitude, time zone**
•**Dehydration**
•**Fatigue, sleep problems**
•**Glaring lights**
•**Perfumes, powerful odors**
•**Stress**

Touch Here for Persistent Back Pain

Daniel C. Cherkin, PhD, is a senior investigator at Group Health Research Institute in Seattle and lead author of a study on lower back pain and massage published in *Annals of Internal Medicine*.

"Oh, my aching back!" If you have ever uttered this common lament—or ever feel tempted to in the future—you will want to know about the surprising results of a recent study. Participants included 401 patients, mostly middle-aged women, who had been suffering for at least three months from chronic low-back pain with no identified cause.

Patients were randomly assigned to receive either "usual care" (the standard treatment doctors typically recommend, including painkillers, anti-inflammatories and/or muscle relaxants) or hour-long massages once per week for 10 weeks. Massage recipients got either the commonly available relaxation massage (also called Swedish massage), which aims to produce an overall sense of relaxation…or structural massage, which uses specialized techniques to alleviate musculoskeletal problems that can contribute to back pain (for instance, by lengthening constricted muscles and mobilizing restricted joints).

Results: After 10 weeks, 36% to 39% of patients in the massage groups reported that their back pain was "much better or gone," versus only 4% of patients in the usual-care group. Also, massaged patients reported spending fewer days in bed, being more active and using less medication than usual-care patients.

Surprising: Contrary to expectations, researchers found that relaxation massage was just as effective as the more specialized structural massage at relieving pain and improving patients' ability to function normally. While the benefits of massage began to decrease after treatment ended, improvement was still evident six months later.

Bottom line: Massage is a generally safe therapy that can be used alone or as a supplement to other treatments for chronic low-back pain. Though relaxation massage typically is not covered by health insurance, some policies do cover structural massage, which is considered similar to physical therapy.

Get Rid of Back Pain in Just 7 Minutes a Day

Gerard Girasole, MD, an orthopedic spine surgeon at The Orthopaedic & Sports Medicine Center in Trumbull, Connecticut. He is coauthor, with Cara Hartman, CPT, a Fairfield, Connecticut–based certified personal trainer, of *The 7-Minute Back Pain Solution: 7 Simple Exercises to Heal Your Back without Drugs or Surgery in Just Minutes a Day.*

O f the 30 million Americans who suffer from low back pain, only about 10% of the cases are caused by conditions that require surgery, such as pinched nerves or a slipped disk.

For the overwhelming majority of back pain sufferers, the culprit is tight, inflamed muscles.

Surprising: This inflammation usually is not caused by strain on the back muscles themselves, but rather a strain or injury to the spine—in particular, to one of five "motion segments" in the lower back.

Each segment, which is constructed to bend forward and back and side to side, consists of a disk (the spongy cushion between each pair of spinal vertebrae)…the two vertebrae directly above and below it…and the facets (joints) connecting the vertebrae to the disk.

Unfortunately, the segments' disks or facets can be injured in a variety of ways—by lifting something the wrong way, twisting too far, sitting too long or even sneezing too hard—causing the surrounding muscles to contract in order to protect the spine from further damage.

This contraction and the muscle inflammation that it produces is what causes the intense lower back pain that so many Americans are familiar with.

WHEN BACK PAIN STRIKES

Low back pain caused by inflammation usually subsides on its own within three to six weeks.* However, the healing process can be accelerated significantly by taking over-the-counter *ibuprofen* (Motrin) for several days after injury to reduce inflammation if you don't

*If you suffer from severe back pain or back pain accompanied by fever, incontinence or weakness or numbness in your leg, see a doctor right away to rule out a condition that may require surgery, such as serious damage to disks, ligaments or nerves in the back.

have an ulcer (follow label instructions)…and getting massage therapy to help loosen knotted muscles and increase healing blood flow to them.

Also important: Perform the simple stretching routine described in this article. In my more than 16 years of practice as an orthopedic spine surgeon, it is the closest thing I've found to act as a "silver bullet" for back pain.

How it works: All of the muscles stretched in this routine attach to the pelvis and work in concert to stabilize the spine. Stretching increases blood flow to these specific muscles, thereby reducing the inflammation that leads to painful, tightened back muscles.

GETTING STARTED

In preparation for the back stretch routine described here, it's important to learn a simple approach that systematically stimulates and strengthens your core (abdominal, back and pelvic muscles). This is one of the best ways to protect your spine. Although there are many types of exercises that strengthen the core, abdominal contractions are the easiest to perform.

What to do: Pretend that you have to urinate and then stop the flow—a movement known as a Kegel exercise. Then while lying on your back, place your hands on your pelvis just above your genitals. Now imagine that someone is about to punch you in the stomach, and feel how your lower abdomen tightens protectively.

To do a full abdominal contraction, combine these two movements, holding the Kegel movement while tightening your lower abdomen. Then, continuously hold the full abdominal contraction during all of the stretches described on this page.

7-MINUTE STRETCHING ROUTINE

Do the following routine daily until your back pain eases (start out slowly and gently if you're still in acute pain). Then continue doing it several times a week to prevent recurrences. Regularly stretching these muscles makes them stronger, leaving your lower spine less prone to painful, back-tightening strains.

1. Hamstring wall stretch. Lie face-up on a carpeted floor (or on a folded blanket for

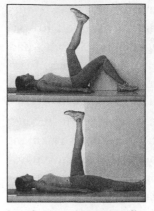

padding), positioning your body perpendicular inside a doorframe. Bend your right leg and place it through the door opening. Bring your buttocks as close to the wall as possible and place the heel of your left foot up against the wall until it is nearly straight. Next, slide your right leg forward on the floor until it's straight, feeling a stretch in the back of your left leg. Hold for 30 seconds. Repeat twice on each side.

2. Knees to chest stretch. Lie on your back with your feet flat on the floor and your

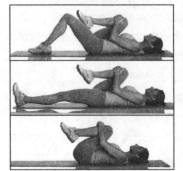

knees bent. Use your hands to pull your right knee to your chest. Next, try to straighten your left leg on the floor. While keeping your right knee held to your chest, continue the stretch for 20 seconds, then switch sides and repeat. Finally, do the stretch by holding both knees to your chest for 10 seconds.

3. Spinal stretch. While on the floor with your left leg extended straight, pull your right

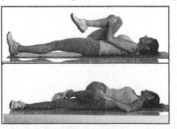

knee to your chest (as in stretch #2), then put your right arm out to the side. Next, use your left hand to slowly pull your right knee toward your left side so that your right foot rests on the back of your left knee. Finally, turn your head toward your right side. Hold for 20 seconds, then reverse the movements and repeat.

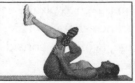

4. Gluteal (buttocks) stretch. Lie on your back with your feet flat on the floor and your knees bent. Cross your right leg over your left, resting your right ankle on your left knee. Next, grab your left thigh with both hands and bring both legs toward your body. Hold for 30 seconds, then switch sides and repeat.

5. Hip flexor stretch. Kneel on your right knee (use a thin pillow for comfort) with your

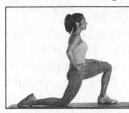

left leg bent 90° in front of you and your foot flat on the floor. Place your right hand on your waist and your left hand on top of your left leg. Inhale and then, on the exhale, lean forward into your right hip, feeling a stretch in the front of your right hip. Hold for 30 seconds, then switch sides and repeat.

6. Quadriceps stretch. While standing, hold on to the back of a sturdy chair with

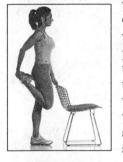

your left hand for balance. Grasp your right foot with your right hand and gently pull your right leg back and up, with your toes pointing upward. Be sure to keep your right knee close to your left leg. Hold for 30 seconds, then switch sides and repeat.

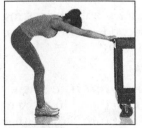

7. Total back stretch. Stand arm's length in front of a table or other sturdy object and lean forward with knees slightly bent so that you can grasp the table edge with both hands. Keep your arms straight and your head level with your shoulders. Hold for 10 seconds.

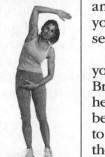

Next, stand up straight with your left hand in front of you. Bring your right arm over your head with elbow bent, then bend your upper body gently to the left. Hold for 10 seconds, then switch sides and repeat.

Photos: Scott Wynn

You Can Conquer Nagging Pain Once and For All

The late Bonnie Prudden, who helped create the President's Council on Youth Fitness in 1956 and has been one of the country's leading authorities on exercise therapy for more than five decades. In 2007, she received the Lifetime Achievement Award from the President's Council on Physical Fitness and Sports. She authored 18 books, including *Pain Erasure*.

C an you imagine living well into your 90s and being able to eliminate virtually all of the aches and pains that you may develop from time to time?

Ninety-seven-year-old Bonnie Prudden, a longtime physical fitness advocate, lived pain free—even though she had arthritis that led to two hip replacements—by using a form of myotherapy ("myo" is Greek for muscle) that she developed more than 30 years ago.

Now: Tens of thousands of patients have successfully used this special form of myotherapy, which is designed to relieve "trigger points" (highly irritable spots in muscles) that develop throughout life due to a number of causes, such as falls, strains or disease.

By applying pressure to these sensitive areas and then slowly releasing it, it's possible to relax muscles that have gone into painful spasms, often in response to physical and/or emotional stress.

A simple process: Ask a partner (a spouse or friend, for example) to locate painful trigger points by applying his/her fingertips to parts of your body experiencing discomfort—or consult a practitioner trained in myotherapy.*

If you're working with a partner, let him know when a particular spot for each body area described in this article is tender.

Pressure should be applied for seven seconds (the optimal time determined by Prudden's research to release muscle tension) each time that your partner locates such a spot.

*To find a practitioner of Bonnie Prudden's myotherapy techniques, go to *www.bonnieprudden.com* or call 800-221-4634. If you are unable to find a practitioner near you, call local massage therapists and ask whether they are familiar with the techniques.

On a scale of one to 10, the pressure should be kept in the five- to seven-point range—uncomfortable but not intolerable.

The relaxed muscles are then gently stretched to help prevent new spasms.

If you prefer to treat yourself: Use a "bodo," a wooden dowel attached to a handle, and a lightweight, metal "shepherd's crook" to locate trigger points and apply pressure. Both tools are available at 800-221-4634, *www.bonnieprudden.com*, for $9 and $39.95, respectively.

For areas that are easy to reach, use the bodo to locate trigger points and then apply pressure to erase them. For spots that are difficult to reach, use the shepherd's crook to find and apply pressure to trigger points.

As an alternative to the specially designed tools, you can use your fingers, knuckles or elbows on areas of the body that can be reached easily. *Common types of pain that can be relieved by this method...* **

SHOULDER PAIN

Finding the trigger point: Lie face down while your partner uses his elbow to gently apply pressure to trigger points that can hide along the top of the shoulders and in the upper back. If you are very small or slender, your partner can use his fingers instead of his elbow.

Place one of your arms across your back at the waist while your partner slides his fingers under your shoulder blade to search for and apply pressure to additional trigger points. Repeat the process on the opposite side.

While still lying face down, bend your elbows and rest your forehead on the backs of your hands. With his hands overlapped, your partner can gently move all 10 of his fingers along the top of the shoulder to locate additional trigger points.

Pain-erasing stretch: The "shrug" is a sequence of shoulder exercises performed four times after myotherapy and whenever shoulder tension builds.

From a standing or sitting position, round your back by dropping your head forward while bringing the backs of your arms together as close as possible in front of your body. Extend both arms back (with your thumbs leading) behind your body while tipping your head back and looking toward the ceiling.

Next, with both arms at your sides, raise your shoulders up to your earlobes, then press your shoulders down hard.

LOW-BACK PAIN

Finding the trigger point: Lie face down while your partner stands to your right and reaches across your body to place his elbow on your buttocks in the area where the left back pocket would appear on a pair of pants. For seven seconds, your partner should slowly apply pressure to each trigger point—not straight down but angled back toward himself.

Repeat on the other side. If the pressure causes slight discomfort, your partner has found the right spot! If not, your partner should move his elbow slightly and try the steps again. Two to three trigger points can typically be found on each buttock.

Pain-erasing stretch: Lie on your left side on a flat surface (such as a bed, table or the floor). Bend your right knee and pull it as close to your chest as possible.

Next, extend your right leg, keeping it aligned with the left leg and about eight inches above it.

Finally, lower the raised leg onto the resting one and relax for three seconds. Perform these steps four times on each leg.

HIP PAIN

Finding the trigger point: The trigger points for hip pain are often found in the gluteus medius, the muscle that runs along either side of the pelvis.

Lie on your side with your knees slightly bent. Using one elbow, your partner should scan for trigger points along the gluteus medius (in the hip area, roughly between the waist and the bottom seam of your underpants) and apply pressure straight down at each sensitive spot for seven seconds.

The same process should be repeated on the opposite side of your body.

Pain-erasing stretch: Lie on your left side on a table with your right leg hanging off the

---

**Check with your doctor before trying this therapy if you have a chronic medical condition or have suffered a recent injury.

side and positioned forward. Your partner should place one hand on top of your waist and the other hand on the knee of the dangling right leg.

This knee should be gently pressed down eight times. The stretch should be repeated on the opposite side.

Strong Hands, Long Life?

Elaine LaLanne, wife of the late Jack LaLanne, is the author or coauthor of numerous books on exercise and health, including the classic *Fitness After 50 Workout*. *JackLalanne.com*

Can our ability to open a jar of pickles or wring out a washcloth give us a greater chance of living longer? That's an implication of recent research published in *British Medical Journal* (BMJ).

Scientists in the UK analyzed data on more than 53,000 people from 14 separate studies, ranking them into four groups based on the strength of their grips.

Findings: Compared with the group that had the strongest hands, those with the weakest grips were 67% more likely to die during the study periods (which ranged from less than five years to more than 20 years). The link between grip strength and longevity was seen not only among seniors, but also in studies in which participants were younger than 60 years old, on average.

This research doesn't necessarily prove that strengthening our hands will prolong our lives—but it well might. Besides, strong hands certainly do make countless daily tasks easier.

When we went looking for grip-building exercises to share with readers, we found a hand workout developed by Jack LaLanne, often called the "godfather of fitness," who passed away at age 96. His widow and coauthor, Elaine LaLanne, said, "Jack did hand exercises every single morning for strength, coordination, dexterity and flexibility."

Here's the LaLanne daily hand workout, which takes about 10 to 15 minutes. All exercises can be done standing or sitting. Why not try them for yourself? (As with any exercise program, get your doctor's OK before beginning. These particular hand exercises may not be appropriate for people with certain medical conditions—for example, carpal tunnel syndrome.)

• **Big squeeze.** Use a rubber ball that fits easily into your palm. Grasp ball with all five fingers of right hand and squeeze as tightly as possible...hold for a count of three...release. Do 10 repetitions (reps), then switch hands. Work your way up to three sets.

• **Hand flexes.** Extend arms straight out in front of you at mid-chest height, palms up, fingers spread. Quickly clench hands into fists, then open again. Do 10 reps as rapidly as possible...then repeat with palms facing down. Work up to three sets.

• **Shake-a-hand.** Hold hands out in front of you and shake them, moving arms all around in whatever manner you like. Continue for one minute...work up to two minutes.

• **Newspaper roll.** Unfold a section of newspaper (try four full sheets to start—if that proves too easy, use eight to 10 sheets). With both hands, grasp the newspaper at one end so that hands are shoulder-width apart. Elbows straight, extend arms in front of you at chest height, palms facing down. Begin rolling up the newspaper, twisting as if wringing out a towel...when you reach the end, reverse the motion to unroll newspaper. Work up to 10 sets.

• **Five to four.** Hold hands in front of you at shoulder height, elbows comfortably bent, palms facing forward, fingers spread wide (as if each hand were indicating the number five). Then bring thumbs across palms (as if indicating the number four)...then extend thumbs again. Do 10 reps at a moderately fast pace. Work up to three sets.

• **Knuckle sandwich.** Hold hands in front of you at shoulder height, elbows comfortably bent, palms facing forward, fingers together and pointing up. Without making a full fist or bending wrists, curl fingers until fingertips touch tops of palms...hold for a count of five...then uncurl fingers. Do 10 reps. Work up to three sets.

• **Spread 'em.** Place hands flat on a desktop or tabletop in front of you, fingers spread as wide as possible. Press down firmly for 10 seconds, then relax. Do three reps.

The Trouble with the New Hip Trend

Ashley William Blom, MD, PhD, professor of orthopedic surgery, University of Bristol School of Clinical Sciences, Bristol, UK, and lead author of a study published in *The Lancet*.

A few years back, many folks with hurting hips were happy to learn that a newer bone-preserving procedure called hip resurfacing could spare them from the more drastic hip replacement.

But: A huge study has now shown that the newer procedure is more likely to lead to problems than the traditional total hip replacement.

Ashley William Blom, MD, lead author of the recent study, weighed in on the results and what they mean for patients contemplating hip surgery.

HIP TALK

In a traditional hip replacement, the femoral head (the bony ball at the top of the thighbone that fits into the hip socket) and femoral neck (the angled piece of bone connecting the head to the main shaft of the thighbone) are completely removed, along with the damaged portion of the hip socket. They are replaced with a ceramic, metal or plastic ball-and-socket mechanism attached to a long stem that is inserted into the thighbone shaft.

In contrast, with hip resurfacing, only superficial layers of the femoral head are removed. The area is then covered with a metal-on-metal cap-and-bearing assembly. Since little bone is removed and no long stem goes into the shaft, resurfacing seems relatively noninvasive. However, resurfacing does require a large incision that cuts and stretches a significant amount of muscle tissue. Resurfacing generally is considered most appropriate for younger, healthier patients who would be expected to recover fairly easily, as some proponents claim it gives better function in more physically demanding patients.

To compare the success rates of these two procedures, Dr. Blom and his colleagues examined data on 434,560 hip operations performed between 2003 and 2011. They analyzed which surgeries ultimately failed and needed to be redone within seven years of the original procedure. Reasons for such failure included unexplained long-term pain, fracture of the femoral neck and/or a negative reaction of the soft tissue to the metal implant.

AND THE WINNER IS...

Almost across the board, resurfacing procedures were more likely to fail—and to do so more quickly—than total replacements.

Among men, the smaller the femoral head, the higher the chance that the resurfacing implant would fail.

Exception: Men with large femoral heads (generally men with large frames) had fairly comparable success rates with resurfacing and with replacement, so Dr. Blom noted that there still may be a place for hip resurfacing among this select group. However, fewer than one-fourth of study participants fell into that category.

Women fared much worse, suffering resurfacing failure rates that were "unacceptably high," Dr. Blom said—up to five times higher than with replacement. Since problems were common even among women with relatively large femoral heads, he now recommends against hip resurfacing for women.

Bottom line: Despite marketing campaigns that use terms like "young and active" to sell the public on the hip-resurfacing trend, it seems as though this is one case in which the old way is better than the new way.

What if you already had hip resurfacing? Dr. Blom said to alert your doctor right away if you develop pain in the hip or leg or difficulty walking, which might signal a fracture or other problem at the surgical site. He also advised seeing your doctor annually—even if you feel fine—so he or she can check for problems that you may not necessarily see or feel. For example, a doctor can tell you definitively whether you have a fracture or a negative reaction to the metal implant.

6

Guilt-Free Pampering

Treat Yourself Like a Goddess

We women are all too prone to exaggerated self-criticism—about our appearance, personalities, accomplishments or whatever. This negative self-talk can drag us down, deflating our self-esteem and even contributing to depression. But: It doesn't have to be this way.

In my work as a therapist, I have seen beautiful transformations take place when women are encouraged to think of themselves not as defective, but as divine—as goddesses! Consider the Greek Athena, the Hindu Shakti, the Roman Diana, the Egyptian Isis or any of innumerable other female divinities, all of whom evoke respect and honor. Envisioning yourself as such a goddess and treating yourself accordingly can help you cast aside habitual self-denunciation. *To pay homage to the spark of divinity within yourself...*

•**Express inner appreciation.** At random times in the day (for instance, when you are waiting at a stoplight or walking the dog), compose a list in your mind about what makes you special—your wisdom, sense of humor, kindheartedness, strong work ethic, toned arms, winning smile. When you have a moment, write down your list of attractive qualities and memorize it. Then, whenever you catch yourself in a self-deprecating thought (I'm so fat that I look terrible in everything I own) or berate yourself for something trivial (I forgot to send my sister a birthday card, I'm a rotten person), mentally review your list of positive characteristics. Let these affirmations become a form of a benediction (a word rooted in the concept "to speak well of").

•**Seek inspiration from goddesses of myth, fiction and history.** Learning the stories of revered female figures can help you

Judy Kuriansky, PhD, is a clinical psychologist and sex therapist on the adjunct faculty of Teachers College, Columbia University in New York City. She is the author of five books, including *The Complete Idiot's Guide to a Healthy Relationship. DrJudy.com*

53

identify qualities that you would like to incorporate as your own. Check out the exercises in the book *A Goddess Is a Girl's Best Friend* by Laurie Sue Brockway.

Examples: To see yourself as lovable and beautiful, evoke the spirit of Venus (the Roman goddess of love) by writing an impassioned love letter to yourself…to let go of workaholism and embrace leisure, try channeling Bast (the Egyptian goddess of play) by singing joyfully in the shower or emulating children at play.

Also helpful: Download and display images of your favorite goddesses to help you visualize your goals.

•**Tout your successes.** It is OK to toot your own horn sometimes, particularly to your partner, friends and others who truly care about you and will celebrate you (rather than people who might become envious). Sharing significant successes ("I finished writing the first draft of my novel!") or even minor ones ("That crossword puzzle was really tough, but I nailed it") reminds you to appreciate your own abilities and allows others to rejoice with you.

•**Accept adulation with grace.** When paid a compliment ("That's a beautiful dress"), do you automatically dismiss or minimize it? Resist the temptation to say, "This old rag?" *Instead:* Simply smile, say thank you and even add an upbeat remark of your own ("I've always liked it, too"), as you let the good feeling of someone else's appreciation wash over you. If you still have trouble with compliments, try picturing yourself on a pedestal as you remind yourself that you deserve to be loved, admired and treated well.

•**Stage a "goddess night."** Ask your partner or best friend to agree to this exercise, where one evening together is totally devoted to pleasing you. For instance, he or she can take you out on the town or prepare an elegant home-cooked dinner…lavish you with compliments and constant attention…present you with a small gift…accompany you on a special activity, such as splurging on orchestra seats at the theater or having a spa day…or even do something as simple as letting you pick the television station. Assure the other person that you will return the favor another

time, and he or she will be that much happier to indulge you.

Spa Indulgences with Proven Health Benefits

Michael Tompkins, RN, LMT, a registered nurse and a licensed massage therapist, is CEO and general manager of Hilton Head Health, a weight loss and wellness resort in South Carolina.

Luxuriating at a spa can make us feel like pampered princesses—but there is no reason to feel guilty about the pleasure. In fact, we're doing ourselves a world of good when we indulge in spa services that have been scientifically proven to promote health and well-being. The benefits include stress reduction, of course, but they go far beyond that.

We spoke with Michael Tompkins, RN, LMT, a registered nurse, licensed massage therapist and CEO and general manager of Hilton Head Health in South Carolina, to discuss the newest research behind health-boosting spa services—and the shift it is bringing in spa clients' expectations. He pointed out that clientele today are more selective, trending toward therapies with demonstrable results…and he cited as prime examples the following four spa services. Each generally is safe, Tompkins confirmed, though it is important to check with your doctor first if you are pregnant or have a medical condition.

Prices vary greatly depending on location and the type of spa you choose, so inquire about prices directly at the facilities you are considering—and ask whether a particular service costs less when done as an add-on to another service. *Consider trying…*

•**Mud therapy.** Certain types of mud contain magnesium and other beneficial minerals that moisturize and nourish the skin and help draw toxins out of pores—which is why mud therapy may ease dermatologic conditions such as acne, eczema and psoriasis.

Therapeutic mud also may help relieve arthritis pain, as several recent studies show.

Evidence: An Israeli study showed that 20-minute mudpack treatments applied to the extremities, neck and back once daily for two weeks reduced stiffness and pain and improved grip strength in people with rheumatoid arthritis, with improvement lasting from one to three months. A Turkish study found that patients with knee osteoarthritis who were given 12 sessions of daily mud therapy experienced improvement in physical function that persisted for three months after treatment.

What to expect: At some spas, you can take an actual mud bath, immersed up to your neck in warm mud. More typically, warm mud is applied directly to body areas that are painful (such as joints) or to areas that you want to draw toxins from, such as the face. The treated area is wrapped in gauze for 20 minutes or so…then the wrapping is removed and the mud rinsed away.

Note: Therapeutic mud usually has a strong sulfur smell, which some people may find unpleasant.

•**Mineral water bath.** The special water used for this treatment is rich in minerals such as magnesium, potassium, calcium, sodium and sulfur, which are thought to have anti-inflammatory, antibacterial and/or moisturizing properties. In addition to research demonstrating benefits for improving the skin condition psoriasis, several recent European studies showed encouraging results from treating osteoarthritis with mineral water baths. For instance, in a study of patients with arthritic knee pain, one group took 30-minute mineral water baths five days a week for four weeks… a second group bathed in tap water. Both groups reported significant improvement on measures of pain, stiffness and physical function—but only in the mineral water group did the benefits persist after three months.

How it is done: You soak some or all of your body (up to the neck) in a tub full of warm mineral water for 15 to 30 minutes.

•**Massage.** A massage not only feels fantastic and leaves you blissfully relaxed, it also loosens tight muscles and releases waste products (such as lactic acid) that can lead to muscle stiffness and soreness. Numerous studies show additional benefits—for instance, massage can help alleviate pain, including chronic low-back pain…reduce blood pressure…boost the immune response and promote healing in patients suffering from burns or cancer…reduce aggression…ease depression…and improve sleep.

There are many types of massage. While some people like intense hands-on pressure, massage does not have to be painful to be therapeutic. *Options…*

•**Swedish massage,** the most popular, combines kneading and long muscle strokes using light to medium pressure.

•**Hot stone massage** uses the warmth of basalt stones to penetrate muscles, loosening them prior to gentle, relaxing tissue manipulation.

•**Shiatsu massage** aims to restore the natural flow of energy to your meridian points through gentle finger and palm pressure.

•**Thai massage** combines rhythmic holds and stretches that promote energy flow while reducing tension.

•**Deep tissue massage** is intense, using maximum pressure to release chronic muscle tension.

•**Athlete's massage** involves intense, constant pressure with targeted stretching.

•**Reflexology.** This therapy is based on the concept that certain areas of the foot correspond to various parts of the body. For instance, the toes are associated with the head and neck…the arch of the foot corresponds to the internal organs…and the ball of the foot corresponds to the chest and lungs. By applying manual pressure to certain zones on the foot, reflexologists aim to remove energy blockages and bring the body into ideal balance. From a Western perspective, studies show that stimulating and massaging the foot can reduce fatigue and stress, promote circulation and strengthen immunity.

Evidence: In a Korean study, middle-aged women were trained to do reflexology on themselves daily for six weeks. By the end of the study, participants showed significant improvement in measures of stress, depression and immune system response, plus reduced systolic blood pressure.

Recommended: If you want a genuine reflexology experience (rather than a simple foot massage), confirm that the spa's reflexologist is certified by the American Reflexology Certification Board or a state certification program.

Treat Yourself to a Personal Retreat

The late Vidya Carolyn Dell'uomo was president, senior coach and consultant at Open to Life Consultancy in Manlius, New York, and a founding member and faculty member at the Kripalu Center for Yoga and Health in Stockbridge, Massachusetts. She held an advanced yoga certification from the Lakulish Yoga Institute in Kayavorohan, India, and had certification training in social psychology, management, Gestalt therapy, body-mind therapy and yoga science.

Music is the silence between the notes, the French composer Claude Debussy said…so the true song is in the "rests."

Yet in our everyday busyness, the fundamental nature of the rest often is overlooked. Our lives become as garbled as a ballad played at top speed, devoid of the pauses so essential to its beauty.

How can we make room in our lives to restore those pauses? One way is to go on a personal retreat. Unlike vacations (which sometimes create more stress than they relieve), a personal retreat provides an opportunity for deep rest and reflection, helping to renew the body, mind, heart and spirit. As life coach Vidya Carolyn Dell'uomo, a founding member of the retreat site Kripalu Center for Yoga and Health in Massachusetts, put it, "Vacations are about external sightseeing, but a personal retreat is about internal sightseeing."

What to expect on a retreat: Centers for retreats usually are located in nonurban areas away from the bustle of everyday life. Though some retreat centers cater to groups (families, corporations), the idea of the personal retreat is to focus on yourself as an individual.

Personal retreats fall into two basic categories—structured and unstructured (also called directed and self-directed). A structured retreat typically includes guided activities, such as yoga classes, meditation, breath work, journal writing and dream boards (a visual representation of hopes and dreams created with pictures and cutouts). Dell'uomo recommended choosing a structured program for your first retreat so that you have some guidance on how to get the most out of the experience. Later, you may wish to try an unstructured retreat.

Consider how much time you can devote to your retreat—a day, several days, a week or more.

Keep in mind: "It takes time to 'settle' —to acclimate to a new pace. By the middle of a longer retreat, a deepening occurs…the retreat takes on a life of its own…and insights arise from a well deep within," Dell'uomo said.

To find a retreat, ask friends for recommendations or surf the Web. [*Editor's note*: An online resource such as *www.RetreatFinder.com* lets you search by location, environment (desert, mountain, rain forest), focus (wellness, arts, women only) and other criteria.] To get a better sense of which retreat would be best for you, identify several possibilities and then call the centers to ask about their programs, accommodations, philosophy and prices.

Retreat costs vary greatly depending on duration, location and activities. Dell'uomo said, "It may not be true, in the case of retreats, that you get what you pay for. Some high-end retreats occur in lush settings with spa facilities, and if pampering is what you are looking for, these may be worth your money. Other retreats, especially those at spiritual centers, may have simpler accommodations and amenities yet provide a guided experience in self-reflection that is worth its weight in gold."

The best part about taking a retreat is what happens afterward. Dell'uomo pointed out, "A personal retreat paves the way for integrating into your daily life the practices that sustain and nourish the peace and balance that we all long for."

Comfort in a Cup: Healing Herbal Teas

Brigitte Mars, adjunct professor of herbal medicine at Naropa University in Boulder, Colorado. She is a professional member of the American Herbalists Guild and author of *Healing Herbal Teas. BrigitteMars.com*

Herbal teas help soothe pain, ease stress and treat disease—more economically and with fewer side effects than drugs.

For convenience: Use tea bags.

For potency: Use loose organic herbs (sold in health-food stores).

Instructions: Boil eight ounces of water. Remove from heat. Stir in one heaping tablespoon of dried herbs or three level tablespoons of fresh herbs. Steep 10 minutes. Remove tea bag or strain off loose herbs. Drink hot or iced. Have two to three cups daily until symptoms subside…then one cup every few days to maintain health.*

CHAMOMILE TEA EASES…

- **Insomnia**
- **Gastrointestinal upset**
- **Inflammation**

How it works: It has mild sedative properties to calm nerves…stimulates production of digestive fluids…and may inhibit metabolism of arachidonic acid, an inflammatory omega-6 fatty acid.

Keep in mind: Steep no longer than three to five minutes to prevent bitterness. Discontinue two weeks before any surgery. Do not use if you are allergic to ragweed, celery or onion or take blood-thinning drugs.**

GINGER TEA EASES…

- **Nausea, motion sickness, morning sickness**
- **Colds and flu**

*Some herbs can interact with drugs or cause allergic reactions. Always consult your doctor before using herbal tea, especially if you have heart disease, diabetes, ulcers, gallbladder problems, a bleeding or seizure disorder, or a kidney or liver disorder, or if you are anticipating surgery.

**Do not use if you are pregnant or breast-feeding.

- **Pain** (sore throat, arthritis, migraine)

How it works: It stimulates secretion of digestive fluids…reduces congestion and inflammation…and bolsters the immune system. It also reduces risk for blood clots.

Keep in mind: Steep it in hot (but not boiling) water. Discontinue two weeks before any surgery. Do not use if you have heartburn, ulcers or gallbladder problems or take blood-thinning or diabetes drugs.

GINSENG TEA EASES…

- **Low energy**
- **Low libido**

How it works: It boosts the immune system…increases the body's resistance to stress…and contains phytosterols (steroid-like plant chemicals) that may promote proper hormone function.

Keep in mind: For best effect, drink between meals. Discontinue two weeks before any surgery. Do not use if you take blood-thinning or diabetes medication…or have a history of breast cancer.**

NETTLE TEA EASES…

- **Arthritis pain**
- **Bloating**
- **Allergies, asthma**

How it works: It reduces inflammation… acts as a diuretic…and may deactivate mast cells (which release histamine, a chemical that provokes mucous membrane hyperactivity).

Keep in mind: It is best to use dried nettle —the fresh plant can cause a stinging rash. Discontinue if it causes gastrointestinal upset. Do not use if you have any problems with blood sugar.**

PASSIONFLOWER TEA EASES…

- **Anxiety**
- **Stress**
- **Drug or alcohol withdrawal**

How it works: It may slow the breakdown of calming neurotransmitters…and it has sedative effects.

**Do not use if you are pregnant or breast-feeding.

Keep in mind: It is slightly bitter, so add honey or agave nectar for a sweeter taste. Do not use with blood-thinning drugs or with sedating medication (sleeping pills, certain antihistamines, or painkillers).**

PEPPERMINT TEA EASES...

- **Stomach upset**
- **Bad breath**

How it works: It increases circulation to the digestive tract...improves flow of digestive fluids...calms intestinal spasms...suppresses mouth chemicals that contribute to bad breath.

Keep in mind: It is safe to use when pregnant or breast-feeding. Do not use if you have a hiatal hernia or gallbladder problems.

**Do not use if you are pregnant or breast-feeding.

Love Your Looks...No Matter What Your Age

Pamela D. Blair, PhD, holistic therapist in private practice, life coach and motivational speaker in Shelburne, Vermont. She coordinated the Institute for Spiritual Development at Wainwright House, a learning center in Rye, New York. *PamBlair.com*

D o you catch your reflection in a mirror and feel shock when you see an "old woman" gazing back, because inside you still feel so young?

Coping with our changing appearance requires looking inward. Coming to rely on who we are rather than what we look like yields profound confidence, strength and self-assurance that often elude younger people. Paradoxically, that self-knowledge creates a magnetism that also is deeply attractive. *To nourish healthy self-acceptance...*

- **Savor each day.** Perhaps more than any other quality, being able to take pleasure in life makes a woman beautiful.

- **Pay attention to your senses.** Really taste the food you eat. Feel the fresh air on your skin as you walk outdoors. Relish the touch of a loved one. Some attractive qualities we tend to associate with youth—eagerness, curiosity, openness—can become stronger with age if we take time to appreciate the world around us.

- **Reexamine your goals.** Does your life now reflect your true values? Or are you investing time in relationships that are no longer fulfilling...activities that are no longer interesting...surroundings that no longer meet your needs?

Each morning, try this affirmation exercise. Say, "I am a woman who..." 10 times, and finish the sentence with a different ending each time, specifying goals you are striving for.

Examples: "I am a woman who is free of back pain...likes a gentle, relaxed pace to her life...has all the financial rewards she wants and needs...takes pleasure in her work."

After several weeks, notice what has shifted in your life. Even if these dreams have not yet come true for you, the power of positive thought can help bring about profound changes in the choices you make and in the way you live.

Example: If I am a woman who is free of back pain, I will choose not to lift that heavy box, and I will ask for help instead. I will choose not to skip yoga class. I will take actions that support who I want to be.

- **Reclaim beauty.** We all know that the media promotes an impossible standard of beauty. A recent study at the University of Missouri-Columbia found that women felt worse about their bodies after viewing photos of models in ads.

We do not need to accept the media's definition of beauty. I've stopped reading magazines that show only young, implausibly perfect models in their articles and ads. These pictures are not real. My former husband was an art director for a major fashion magazine, so I often saw the "before" photos of models with wrinkles, crooked noses and large hips—all of which were airbrushed away.

I am learning to be proud of my wrinkles. They represent laughter, conversation, concern for others and the hard work to become a good writer, mother, therapist, gardener. They are symbols of a beautiful life.

• **Find role models who exemplify a more enlightened beauty.** My idol is the actress Tyne Daly—a little overweight, gray-haired, strong-willed, absolutely beautiful and unapologetically not "young." Many European actresses, such as Helen Mirren and Judi Dench, proudly look their age and remain elegant and desirable. I enjoy watching their films and reading about their personal and professional successes. If they can pursue their dreams and not be ashamed of their aging faces, then so can I.

• **Revisit your beauty rituals.** Valuing inner beauty doesn't mean ignoring your appearance. Decide which maintenance routines are worth keeping and which ones you can let go. By fighting the aging process a little less, you gain time and energy that you can put into other fulfilling pursuits. You also will become more relaxed, which is an attractive quality.

Example: I get manicures and pedicures because they make me feel pampered and cared for. They are a source of energy for me, rather than an energy drain. On the other hand, this past year I chose to stop dying my hair. I have gained many hours, and my skin looks better, too—the natural gray provides a softer contrast than the dyed color did. My choice wouldn't work for everyone. Someone who loves dying her hair should keep doing it.

Also experiment with new styles and products that acknowledge your changing body.

Helpful: Make an appointment with an image consultant to find out which clothing styles and colors complement your skin, hair and body shape now. Find a consultant through the Association of Image Consultants International (651-290-7468, *www.aici.org*).

Cost: $75 to $350 per hour, depending on your location and the extent of services provided.

Alternative: Get a free makeover at a department store cosmetics counter.

Example: I learned to switch to a lighter-consistency foundation and to stop using powder, which can emphasize imperfections in skin. My image consultant also suggested V-necklines to draw attention away from my filled-out chin…and pants that drop gently from my wider hips. I look and feel more elegant.

• **Pace yourself to allow for physical changes.** Your strength may be slightly less, your reaction time a bit longer. I have been doing Pilates exercises, which have increased my muscle strength, bone density and energy as well as decreased my arthritis pain.

• **Increase your serenity by taking a meditative approach.** Before you start your day, sit quietly and visualize what you need to accomplish that day. Pick no more than three major tasks, and go about them with full attention.

Once you've completed those tasks, you can add one or two more. Notice how much calmer and more graceful you feel than when you race around trying to cross 20 items off your to-do list yet give them all short shrift. Enjoy the alertness that comes from being fully present with one task at a time. Your increasing serenity will radiate outward, assuredly making you feel and look more beautiful.

How a Quick Massage Can Help You Live Longer

Mark Tarnopolsky, MD, PhD, professor in the departments of pediatrics and medicine, McMaster University, Ontario, Canada.

No one wants to be overweight, have diabetes or grow old prematurely. Well, a new study shows that there's a simple strategy that may help prevent all three that is actually quite fun and relaxing.

A massage might do the trick!

This is not about the expensive, hour-long massage—the latest research shows that an inexpensive massage lasting just 10 minutes can be beneficial.

MASSAGING YOUR MUSCLES TO FIGHT DISEASE

Researchers were interested in studying massage immediately after exercise for two reasons. For one thing, practically speaking, that's a common time for people to get a massage, since many people say that massage helps reduce muscle soreness from exercise. Another reason is that, biologically, it's easier to measure differences in the effect of massage on cells after exercise, because exercise puts the body into a state of temporary stress.

Volunteers in the study included 11 healthy, active men in their 20s who provided a bit of muscle tissue from one thigh for a baseline biopsy. Then researchers had the volunteers do 70 minutes of fast-paced cycling on a stationary bike. The volunteers rested for 10 minutes and then had a 10-minute massage on one thigh only. Immediately after the massage, researchers took second muscle biopsies, but this time from both thighs in order to compare massaged tissue versus nonmassaged tissue. Two and a half hours after the second biopsies, the volunteers underwent a third set of biopsies on both thighs to capture any changes that might have occurred a bit later after their massages.

To learn about the findings, we spoke with Mark Tarnopolsky, MD, PhD, a professor of medicine and head of neuromuscular and neurometabolic disease at McMaster University in Canada, who was a coauthor of the study published in *Science Translational Medicine*.

STOP THE DAMAGE!

Dr. Tarnopolsky said that the researchers found two very interesting differences in the muscles that had been massaged...

A gene pathway that causes muscle inflammation was "dialed down" in these muscles both immediately after the massage and 2.5 hours after the massage. (Specific genes can be present in our tissues but not always active.) Dr. Tarnopolsky said that this is helpful knowledge because muscle inflammation is a contributor to delayed-onset muscle soreness, so it confirms biologically what we've always believed through anecdotal observation—a post-exercise massage can help relieve muscle soreness.

Conversely, another sort of gene was "turned on" by the massage—this is a gene that increases the activity of mitochondria in muscle cells. You probably know that mitochondria are considered the "power packs" of our muscles for their role in creating usable energy. Now, it's true that better mitochondrial functioning has been shown by other studies to help decrease insulin resistance (a key risk factor for type 2 diabetes) and obesity and even to slow aging. When asked about whether or not it's a stretch to link post-exercise massage to these benefits, Dr. Tarnopolsky said that it's not unreasonable—there is a potential connection, and future research will need to be done to confirm it.

TREAT YOURSELF TO MASSAGE

The massage type that Dr. Tarnopolsky and his colleagues used was a standard combination of three techniques that are commonly used for post-exercise massage—effleurage (light stroking)...petrissage (firm compression and release)...and stripping (repeated longitudinal strokes). It's easy to find massage therapists in spas, salons, fitness centers and private practices who use these techniques. Or you could ask your spouse or a friend to try some of these moves on you (even if his or her technique isn't perfect) because there's a chance that it could provide the benefits, said Dr. Tarnopolsky—he just can't say for sure, since that wasn't studied.

Dr. Tarnopolsky studied massage only after exercise, so that's when he would recommend getting one, but it's possible that massaging any muscles at any time may have similar benefits—more research will need to be done to find out.

Remember, you don't have to break the bank on a prolonged 60-minute massage—a simple 10- or 20-minute rubdown (which usually cost $10 to $40) can do the trick.

Give Yourself a Massage!

Paula Koepke, CMT, a massage therapist at the University of California, San Francisco Osher Center for Integrative Medicine, and an instructor at the McKinnon Body Therapy Center in Oakland, California. *Paula Koepke.MassageTherapy.com*

Massage is far more than a mere luxury. It may reduce the stress that contributes to heart disease and digestive disorders…relieve pain by manipulating pressure points that relax muscles…and raise levels of mood-boosting brain chemicals. Good news: You can take your health into your own hands—literally—with simple self-massage techniques.

What to do: Always apply firm but comfortable pressure, repeating each sequence of motions for three to five minutes. Unless noted, techniques can be done while sitting or lying down. Use scented lotion or oil if desired—lavender and rose are calming…peppermint and rosemary are stimulating.

SINUS OR TENSION HEADACHE

• **Lying on your back, place the fingertips of both hands in the center of your forehead**…stroke outward toward the temples…make 10 small slow circles over the temples. Move fingertips to the cheeks, where the jaw hinges…make 10 small slow circles there.

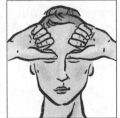

• **Place the pads of your thumbs just below each upper eye ridge (near the brow),** where the ridge meets the bridge of the nose, and press up toward your forehead for 10 seconds. In small increments, move thumbs along the eye ridges toward the outer edges of eyes, pressing for several seconds at each stopping point.

Caution: Always press upward on the bony ridge, not into the eye socket.

• **With fingertips, make small circles all over the scalp for 30 seconds as if washing hair.** Then place fingertips at the back of the neck and make 10 small slow circles at the base of the skull.

STOMACH UPSET OR CONSTIPATION

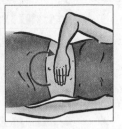

• **Lying on your back, place one hand flat on your abdomen (over or under your clothing) just above your navel.** Pressing gently but firmly, slowly move your hand clockwise to circle the navel.

NECK AND/OR SHOULDER PAIN

• **Sitting, reach your left hand over your right shoulder until it touches above the shoulder blade.** With fingertips, firmly knead muscles, focusing on any sore spots. Repeat on other side.

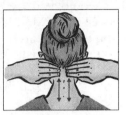

• **Sitting, place fingertips of both hands on the back of the neck at the base of the skull.** Pressing firmly, move fingers up and down along the sides of the vertebrae. To protect major blood vessels, do not massage front or sides of the neck.

FOOT SORENESS

• **Sitting, place your left ankle on your right knee.** Grasp the left foot with your right hand and slowly rotate the foot at the ankle three times in each direction. Then use your fingers to gently rotate toes, one at a time, three times in each direction. Repeat on the other side.

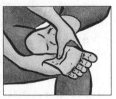

• **Sitting, place your left ankle on your right knee and cradle the left foot in both hands.** With thumbs, make five small slow circles—first on the instep…then the ball of the foot…heel…and pad of each toe. Repeat on your other foot.

Bonus: Performing foot massage for 10 minutes nightly may promote health overall.

Theory of reflexology: "Reflex points" on the feet are linked to various body systems and organs, which benefit from tactile stimulation.

Massage illustrations by Shawn Banner

Why We Need to Watch TV Reruns

Jaye L. Derrick, PhD, assistant professor, social psychology at the University of Houston in Texas, and author of a study on the effects of watching TV reruns published in *Social Psychological & Personality Science.*

Quiz: Plopping down in front of the tube to watch reruns of a favorite show...

A) Turns you into a zoned-out zombie.

B) Is fun but essentially a waste of time.

C) Rejuvenates self-control.

Would you be surprised if the correct answer is C? Well, it's true, according to intriguing new research. *Some background info...*

Psychologists know that it takes work to control one's thoughts, moods and behaviors. Since self-control is not limitless, this "effortful self-control" depletes a finite resource, leaving less self-control available for whatever tasks one might face next. Self-control can be replenished by positive social interactions (such as a nice chat with a friend or a hug from your honey). But social interactions also can be risky—because when things go wrong (for instance, an argument erupts), self-control can wind up being depleted even further.

So for the new study, researchers investigated whether "social surrogacy"—in the form of interaction with a favorite, familiar, fictional world—could replenish flagging self-control. *The study included two separate components...*

Part 1. Participants were asked to write about a recent trip. Half of them were allowed to write what they wanted, which was easy...but the other half were restricted to words that did not contain the letters "a" or "i," which required concentrated effort and thus depleted self-control. Then the groups were reshuffled and assigned a second writing task. Half wrote a list of items in their rooms (a neutral activity)...the other half wrote about a favorite TV show (to trigger feelings associated with social surrogacy). Next, all participants worked on word puzzles, then rated their levels of negative feelings such as anger, dejection and sadness.

Results: Among participants whose self-control had initially been depleted by the restricted writing task, those who wrote about favorite fictional TV characters did better on the word puzzles and reported fewer negative feelings—suggesting that their self-control reserves had been replenished—than those who simply listed household items.

Part 2. Volunteers kept daily diaries for two weeks, noting when they encountered situations that required them to exercise self-control over their thoughts or moods. They also recorded when they reread a beloved book or watched a familiar favorite TV episode or film (the social surrogacy situation)... and when they read a new book, watched a new episode of a show they liked or watched whatever happened to be on TV. In addition, they rated the intensity levels of their negative moods.

Analysis: When participants had to exert a lot of self-control, they were more likely to reread a favorite book or watch a favorite rerun afterward—an indication that they were subconsciously seeking the rejuvenating comfort of a familiar fictional world. Those who did not use this social surrogacy to replenish self-control were more likely to report negative moods afterward.

Bottom line: Of course, no one is suggesting that we spend all our free time playing couch potato while ignoring chores, work, family and other responsibilities. After all, a healthy lifestyle must include interactions with other live humans as well as regular physical activity. But it is comforting to know that there's a perfectly good reason to curl up with a well-loved book or settle down to watch a favorite flick or TV show when we're feeling depleted and need a restorative boost.

Feel-Good Fashionable Shoes

Johanna S. Youner, DPM, a leading cosmetic foot surgeon and attending podiatric physician, New York-Presbytarian Hospital, New York City. *HealthyFeet NY.com*

Many shoe companies seem to scarcely consider the natural shape of a woman's foot when they design those tiny, triangular toe boxes and too-high heels. But you can find stylish shoes that won't cause potentially crippling foot deformities or lead to chronic back pain by forcing your hips, knees and ankles out of proper alignment. *What to look for…*

•**High, wide toe box.** If the top of your second toe (often the longest and most prone to arthritis) presses against the top of the shoe, the toe box is too shallow…if toes feel squeezed, the box is too narrow.

Elegant option: An oblique (angled) toe box—longer at the big toe than the little toe—looks stylish and is roomier than a pointy one.

•**Toe coverage.** Showing a bit of toe cleavage looks sexy—but a shoe that barely covers the toes does not stabilize the foot enough, allowing the foot to roll inward or outward. The more the shoe covers the top of the foot, the more support it generally provides.

•**The right heel height.** Heels that force your feet forward are too high…shoes without heels (such as ballet flats) provide no arch support.

Ideal heel: One to two inches high. If you must wear higher heels on occasion, minimize the time spent standing or walking in them.

•**Cushioned insole.** This eases pressure on the ball of the foot. If you feel every pebble underfoot, add an insert, such as Superfeet GO Premium Pain Relief Full Length Insoles ($69.95, 800-634-6618, *www. superfeet.com*).

Brands of foot-friendly, stylish shoes: Dansko, Ecco, Mephisto, Munro, Prada, Rockport, Taryn Rose.

Sweet Talk: Chocolate Helps You Stay Slim

Beatrice A. Golomb, MD, PhD, is a professor of medicine at the University of California, San Diego School of Medicine and lead author of study on chocolate consumption and body mass published in *Archives of Internal Medicine.*

Chocoholics now have one more reason to cheer—because in addition to being rich in heart-healthy antioxidants, this sweet treat may make it easier to keep weight under control, a new study suggests. *Here's the skinny…*

For the study, about 1,000 women and men answered a food questionnaire indicating, among other things, how many times per week they typically consumed chocolate. Weight and height measurements also were taken to calculate body mass index (BMI).

Findings: Participants who ate chocolate more often consumed more calories and saturated fat overall (and exercised about the same amount), yet had a lower average BMI than those who ate chocolate less frequently. What was the magnitude of this difference? Well, for instance, people who indulged in chocolate five times weekly had a BMI of about one point lower—which translates to a body weight of about five to eight pounds less, depending on height—than people who never consumed chocolate.

Fascinating implication: These findings challenge the age-old principle that calorie count is all that really matters for weight control, suggesting instead that our bodies may not treat all calories the same way. One possible explanation for chocolate's slenderizing effects is that certain antioxidant polyphenols in cocoa may favorably influence metabolism by increasing the energy that cells make.

This study looked at the frequency of chocolate consumption, not at the amount or type of chocolate eaten. Still, moderation is advisable, researchers suggested…and previous studies have shown that dark chocolate has particularly positive effects on blood pressure, cholesterol levels and insulin sensitivity. Researchers hope to conduct a randomized clinical trial to further investigate chocolate's potential metabolic benefits—provided they're able to find a control group of people willing to forgo chocolate for the good of science.

Indulge in the Dessert-for-Breakfast Diet…and Lose Weight!

Daniela Jakubowicz, MD, is a former professor of medicine and endocrinology at Virginia Commonwealth University and is now at the Wolfson Medical Center at Tel Aviv University in Israel.
Hannah El-Amin, RD, LD, is a dietitian, certified diabetes educator and trained intuitive eating specialist. *NutritionThatFits.com*

Wasn't it a thrill when a recent study revealed that eating dessert with breakfast could help people lose lots of weight? Whether you want to drop just a few pounds or a whole bunch, the dessert-for-breakfast diet can help. *First, a review of the research for those who missed it…*

In the study, overweight or obese adults were put on diets, with women eating 1,400 calories per day and men eating 1,600 calories per day. Lunches and dinners for all participants were mostly lean meats and salads. But participants were divided into two groups, and the groups differed when it came to their breakfasts. One group ate a small, low-carb breakfast of just 300 calories (typically bacon, eggs and coffee). The other group ate a large, high-protein, high-carb breakfast of 600 calories that usually included a chicken breast or tuna filet sandwich…a glass of milk…and a 150-to-200-calorie dessert, such as chocolate, cookies, cake, ice cream, mousse or donuts.

For the first 16 weeks, participants had to stick strictly to their diets—and both groups lost 33 pounds, on average. For the next 16 weeks, participants were encouraged to continue dieting but were told that they could succumb to cravings if they felt like they needed to. Results at week 32: Members of the small, low-carb breakfast group had regained 22 pounds, on average…while those in the large, high-protein, high-carb breakfast group had dropped another 15 pounds.

Reasons: Daniela Jakubowicz, MD, the study leader and a metabolic disorders specialist currently at the Wolfson Medical Center at Tel Aviv University in Israel, explained that a substantial morning meal shifts your body from the energy-conserving state of sleep to the calorie-burning state of day. She outlined the hormonal factors that allow you to feel satisfied, not famished, even as you lose weight on the dessert-for-breakfast diet…

●**Food eaten early in the morning**—usually before 9 am—reduces levels of ghrelin (a hormone that increases hunger) to a greater extent than food eaten later in the day.

●**The morning dessert raises levels of the feel-good neurotransmitter serotonin,** fending off carbohydrate cravings. What's more, sweets and other high-carb foods cause ghrelin to drop faster than other types of foods.

●**Cortisol, a hormone that helps convert protein to energy, is naturally high in the morning.** Eating enough protein at breakfast increases energy expenditure…helps keep hunger at bay all morning…and prevents your body from using its own muscle proteins for fuel (as happens to those who skip breakfast).

●**The body is more sensitive to insulin early in the day.** When you eat carbs in the morning, insulin more readily facilitates the transport of glucose from these foods to the muscles for use as energy. If you consume these foods at night when insulin is less efficient, however, they get stored as body fat.

To help you apply this research to your daily life, we asked dietitian Hannah El-Amin, RD, for some tasty morning menus that include dessert. Below are her inspiring ideas. Each breakfast provides about 500 to 600 calories… about 55 to 65 grams of carbohydrate…about 35 to 50 grams of protein…and, of course, a sweet treat.

CHOCOLATE-BERRY BREAKFAST

●**Omelet:** 4 egg whites or ½ cup egg substitute filled with chopped spinach and mushrooms, to taste, and 1 Tablespoon crumbled feta cheese

- **2 lean turkey sausage links**
- **2 slices sprouted-grain toast spread with 2 pats butter**
- **1 cup sliced strawberries tossed with 1 Tablespoon mini dark chocolate chips**

MILKSHAKE MORNING MEAL

- **Wrap:** *2 ounces turkey and ¼ cup hummus wrapped in a whole-wheat tortilla*
- **Milkshake:** ¾ cup low-fat milk or soy milk blended with ½ cup yogurt, ½ frozen banana and ½ Tablespoon peanut butter

NUTTY CANDY-APPLE BREAKFAST

- **Toasted whole-wheat English muffin** topped with 1 ounce reduced-fat cream cheese, 2 ounces smoked salmon and 1 teaspoon capers
- **4 egg whites or ½ cup egg substitute,** seasoned to taste and scrambled
- **1 cup soy milk**
- **1 sliced apple sprinkled with cinnamon** and dipped in 1½ Tablespoons almond butter mixed with 1 Tablespoon honey

---

Herbal Baths Detox Your Whole Body

Mao Shing Ni, PhD, DOM (doctor of Oriental medicine), LAc (licensed acupuncturist), is director and a professor of Chinese medicine and cofounder of Yo San University in Santa Monica and cofounder of Tao of Wellness, an acupuncture and Chinese medicine clinic in Santa Monica, Pasedena and Newport Beach, California. He is the author of 12 books, including *Secrets of Longevity: Dr. Mao's 8-Week Program: Simple Steps that Add Years to Your Life.* TaoOfWellness.com

---

Soaking in a hot bath feels fabulous, of course. But did you know that it helps draw toxins out of the body if you put certain herbs and other natural substances in the tub? We asked Mao Shing Ni, PhD, DOM, LAc, author of *Secrets of Longevity: Dr. Mao's 8-Week Program: Simple Steps that Add Years to Your Life,* to share his personal recipe for an herbal bath that uses essential oils or fresh or dried herbs to cleanse you inside and out. *It includes…*

- **Eucalyptus and wintergreen,** which help open the pores so toxins can be more easily expelled through the skin… and which have antibacterial properties.
- **Cinnamon and fennel,** which increase circulation, transporting nutrients and oxygen more efficiently to muscles and organs.
- **Epsom salts (magnesium sulfate),** which help muscles eliminate lactic acid, a by-product of muscle metabolism that causes soreness and cramping.

For best results, Dr. Mao recommended taking an herbal bath daily. If your water contains chlorine (as does the water in many municipalities), consider buying a faucet-mounted filter to eliminate it, since chlorine dries out the skin. Before drawing your bath, rinse away any detergent residue in your tub. Fill the tub as high as you like with moderately hot water (100°F to 105°F). *Then…*

- **Use equal amounts of eucalyptus, wintergreen, cinnamon and fennel.** If you opt for essential oils (which is easiest, Dr. Mao noted), use five drops of each…for fresh herbs, use one tablespoon of each, mixed together and placed inside a tea ball…for dried herbs, use one teaspoon of each, mixed together and placed inside a reusable tea bag or drawstring cheesecloth bag. Add the oils or herbs to the bathwater, then add one cup of Epsom salts. Allow everything to steep for at least 10 minutes. (You can leave the tea ball or fabric bag in the tub while you soak.)
- **Soak in the herbal bath for 15 to 20 minutes.** Don't stay in too long, though, or your skin will dehydrate. (If your fingertips start to wrinkle, it is past time to get out, Dr. Mao noted.)

Herbal baths generally are safe for everyone. However, people with certain medical conditions (high or low blood pressure, circulatory problems, heart disease, obesity, pregnancy) should get their doctor's OK first because any type of extended hot bath could cause blood pressure to spike and then drop. People with diabetes who have numbness from nerve damage should take special care to make sure that the bath water is not too hot. Women with vulvodynia (chronic genital pain) may benefit from warm baths with just the Epsom salts, since the herbs might irritate their ultrasensitive tissues.

Easy, Soothing Treatment for Pelvic Pains—and Other Private Parts

Laurie Steelsmith, ND, a naturopathic physician and acupuncturist based in Honolulu and author of *Natural Choices for Women's Health*.

An unusual form of gynecological health treatment is "gathering steam" around the country—pelvic steam baths, also known by the catchier name, vaginal steam baths. While calling it a vaginal steam bath is definitely attention-getting, it is a misnomer, says Laurie Steelsmith, ND, a naturopathic physician and acupuncturist and author of *Natural Choices for Women's Health*. It's not the vagina, an internal structure, that is the focus but rather the outer genital area, the vulva.

IT HELPS LOTS OF PROBLEMS

Dr. Steelsmith is a fan of pelvic steam baths to bring relief for a number of troublesome complaints, among them to relieve chronic vulvar pain (vulvodynia or vulvar vestibulitis)…muscle spasms (vaginismus)…post-childbirth discomfort, including from episiotomy incision…or following a biopsy in the area. The baths soften and loosen the pelvic muscles, which helps make sex more comfortable for some women, including after childbirth. And there's more. Pelvic steam baths help with vaginitis and yeast infections and to heal trauma to the area.

Dr. Steelsmith urges patients with any of these complaints to consider giving this therapy a try, describing the feeling it gives as "nourishing and cozy." Some spas offer pricey pelvic steam baths, but you can do them easily at home, says Dr. Steelsmith. *Here's how…*

• **Boil four cups of water.** You can use the water plain, but many people like to add herbs or a little essential oil.

If you want to use herbs, you should boil the water for 10 to 15 minutes with the herbs in it. (Use a covered pot to minimize evaporation.) Herbs that are popular for the baths include oregano and basil. For a combination that is both soothing and nourishing, Dr. Steelsmith says to mix equal parts of dried chamomile, calendula (marigold), lavender and red clover.

If you prefer oil, add a few drops of a relatively gentle one (she suggests lavender, which is not likely to be irritating—or, if you have a yeast infection, tea tree oil) to the water after it boils. Avoid harsh oils such as camphor or eucalyptus.

• **Pour your brew into a stainless steel bowl,** and place it under a slatted patio chair in which you can sit wearing no underwear and with your pelvic area exposed to the steam.

A second option—empty most of the water out of a toilet by turning its water supply off and then flushing it. Then put the bowl of hot water in the toilet (make sure the rim of the bowl is above the level of any remaining toilet water) and sit on the toilet seat. This allows the pelvic muscles and floor to relax completely, says Dr. Steelsmith, which improves blood circulation and therefore healing. (Note: Wrap your lower body in a towel to hold the vapors in and capture the steam more efficiently.)

• **Remain over the steam for 15 minutes, no more.** Do this twice a day to treat infections or an episiotomy incision… for all other purposes, do once a day until the problem has resolved.

There's only one safety concern, but it is important (if a little obvious). Make sure you are not burning yourself—the temperature should be what you find comfortable, which typically will be reached 10 minutes or so after boiling.

7

Healing Sleep

Why Women Don't Sleep Well

Have you ever felt frustrated watching a man sleep like a baby while you tossed and turned? Do the strategies that used to help you sleep no longer seem to work? Blame biology, at least in part.

As early as adolescence, gender-based differences in physiology and lifestyle make sleep disorders far more common in women than in men. Because these factors change over time, a woman's sleep problems also change—usually for the worse. So it is no surprise that a 2007 poll from the National Sleep Foundation reported that 67% of American women frequently experience sleep problems.

Fortunately, once you understand what triggers your sleep problems, you can take steps toward a better night's rest.

THE CHILDBEARING YEARS

Some women don't need a calendar to remind them when their period is due. A group of symptoms called premenstrual syndrome (PMS)—including breast tenderness, headaches and joint and muscle pains—can cause sufficient discomfort to interfere with rest. A more severe form is premenstrual dysphoric disorder (PMDD), which can cause insomnia, depression, anxiety and fatigue.

Polycystic ovary syndrome is an endocrine disorder in which the ovaries are enlarged and have multiple cysts. Symptoms include infrequent or irregular periods, weight gain, excessive hair growth, prediabetes and infertility. About 30% to 40% of women with this syndrome experience sleep apnea, in which breathing repeatedly stops during sleep. Sleep apnea causes persistent fatigue and raises a person's risk for cardiovascular disease by increasing blood pressure and decreasing oxygen going to the heart.

Meir H. Kryger, MD, professor of medicine (pulmonary) and clinical professor of nursing at Yale School of Medicine in Connecticut and staff of VA Connecticut Health System. The author of *A Woman's Guide to Sleep Disorders* he has been researching and treating women's sleep problems for more than 25 years.

During pregnancy, the quality of sleep worsens for more than 80% of women. The uterus presses on the bladder (so you wake up often to urinate) and on the stomach (causing heartburn that can keep you awake). Pregnant women also are prone to restless legs syndrome (RLS), an irresistible urge to move the legs, which interferes with sleep.

Sleep disturbances worsen after the baby is born, thanks to nighttime feedings. For the 10% to 15% of women who develop postpartum depression in response to the hormonal fluctuations that follow childbirth, sleeplessness often accompanies depression.

MIDLIFE AND BEYOND

The transition to menopause can be brief or may last as long as seven years. During this stage, called perimenopause, periods become irregular. Due to fluctuating hormone levels, many women experience hot flashes and night sweats caused by dilating blood vessels. These rapid changes in body temperature can awaken women repeatedly.

Menopause typically occurs between ages 48 and 55. One in two postmenopausal women experience a sleep disorder, such as sleep apnea or RLS, while nearly two in three have insomnia at least a few nights each week. One culprit is excess weight, particularly in the neck area. The average woman gains eight pounds after menopause, increasing her risk for sleep apnea.

Another sleep-disturbing factor may be the worry that accompanies caregiving, as women in midlife assume responsibility for aging parents and/or ailing husbands.

Advancing age increases a woman's risk for arthritis, diabetes, cardiovascular disease, depression and other chronic conditions. In addition to the discomforts of the diseases themselves, the medications used to treat such conditions can affect sleep.

FOR BETTER SLUMBER...

The good news: Several simple steps can yield big improvements.

● **Eat light—and early—in the evening.** A heavy, spicy or late-night dinner may trigger heartburn that keeps you awake.

Better: A light dinner two to four hours before bedtime. Limit beverages to avoid middle-of-the-night trips to the toilet.

● **Skip the buzz.** Limit caffeinated beverages to two per day, both before lunch. Have no more than one alcoholic drink per evening, at least three to four hours before bed. When you drink too much or too late, your blood alcohol level drops in the middle of the night, causing brain arousal that wakes you up.

● **Quit smoking.** Many smokers wake at night when blood levels of nicotine fall.

● **Argue in the morning (or not at all).** Evenings should be free from confrontations, strenuous workouts and heart-stopping action films that rev you up when you need to wind down.

Exception: Sex, which promotes sound sleep.

● **Avoid evening naps.** Nap only in the afternoon—and for no more than 45 minutes—to minimize disruptions of your nighttime sleep cycle.

● **Create a relaxing bedtime ritual.** Light reading or soothing music tells your brain it's almost bedtime. A warm bath is especially good because raising the body temperature promotes deep sleep.

● **Don't push back your bedtime.** Your body clock works best when bedtimes and awakening times are consistent.

● **Don't lie there staring at the clock if you can't sleep—get up and do something boring.** Tossing and turning is futile and frustrating. Fold some laundry or read something dull until you feel sleepy.

● **Get help for hormonal problems.** Consult your doctor if you suffer from PMS, PMDD or hot flashes.

● **Don't suffer in silence.** Talk to your doctor if your sleep disturbances are due to illness, stress or the side effects of drugs.

● **See a sleep specialist if you have insomnia more than three times per week for more than a month...if you think you have RLS... or if reports of your snoring and gasping lead you to suspect sleep apnea.** You may need an overnight evaluation in a sleep clinic. Your doctor can provide a referral.

Can't Sleep? A Pill Is Not the Answer

Paul Glovinsky, PhD, clinical director of the Capital Region Sleep/Wake Disorders Center in Albany, New York, adjunct professor at the City College of the City University of New York and clinical psychologist who specializes in sleep problems in a private practice in New York City. Dr. Glovinsky is coauthor, with Arthur Spielman, PhD, of *The Insomnia Answer: A Personalized Program for Identifying and Overcoming the Three Types of Insomnia.*

Insomnia has long been known to make people miserable, but researchers have discovered that it can also increase your risk for serious conditions such as high blood pressure, heart disease, diabetes—and even increase your risk of dying.

Important recent finding: People with persistent sleep problems were three times more likely to die (of any cause) over a 19-year period than those who slept well.

So what's the best way to eliminate sleep problems? For years, doctors have prescribed sleeping pills for people who are plagued by insomnia despite the drugs' potential side effects, such as next-day grogginess, dizziness, nausea and confusion.

Latest development: Many sleep experts now say that a nondrug approach—cognitive behavioral therapy for insomnia (CBT-I)—is the "gold standard."

In fact, CBT-I, which involves counseling sessions to help insomnia sufferers change how they think about sleep, is considered to be more effective than medication for long-term relief, according to the American Academy of Sleep Medicine.

A BAD HABIT

The majority of insomnia sufferers attempt to deal with sleeplessness by adopting routines such as watching TV in bed or napping during the day. However, napping answers the body's desire to sleep at the wrong time. Unfortunately, these practices actually perpetuate insomnia, and it becomes a habit.

The good news: Insomnia can be overcome. Key components of CBT-I…

TIMING IS EVERYTHING

You can't make sleep happen. But you can let it happen by cooperating with your body to "catch the wave" of sleep.

Here's why: Your body needs and wants to sleep—it's a natural drive, like hunger and thirst. The longer you go without sleep, the stronger the drive becomes.

Your body also goes through a daily cycle. Though it may seem surprising, alertness builds throughout the day and peaks in the evening just before sleep. As alertness then winds down, sleep drive ramps up.

When these mechanisms work together, a night's sleep satisfies our sleep need. We stay asleep as long as our alertness cycle remains low, and as the cycle begins to rise, we wake up refreshed.

With insomnia, the rhythms fall out of sync. *To best address this problem…*

THINK BETTER THOUGHTS

CBT-I teaches insomnia sufferers that it becomes a self-fulfilling prophecy if they believe they can't sleep. *Thoughts to counter…*

Thought 1: I need my seven (or eight or whatever) hours, or I'll be a wreck tomorrow.

Fact: While people feel and perform better after a good night's sleep, most function surprisingly well after much less—the first three hours of sleep are the deepest and most restorative.

Thought 2: I can't stand lying awake endlessly like this.

Fact: Insomnia is unpleasant but hardly unbearable. You've survived it before and can do it again.

OTHER STEPS THAT HELP

People who undergo CBT-I are also advised to follow well-known insomnia-fighting strategies, such as not consuming caffeine in any form, including coffee or tea, after early afternoon and not drinking alcohol in the evening, which leads to problems staying asleep later in the night. Other steps include going to bed at the same time each night, following a relaxing routine (no stimulating TV programs or Web surfing at least one hour before bedtime)…and using the bedroom only for sleep and sex. *Also helpful…*

• **Do not nap in the evening, even if you're exhausted.** This interferes with your sleep drive. If sleepiness peaks too early in the evening—for example, your eyes start to close while you're reading or watching TV—get up and walk around.

• **Get up after 20 minutes in bed if you're not yet asleep.** Stay up (read or do chores) until you feel drowsy. If you return to bed and still can't sleep, get up again.

GET PROFESSIONAL HELP

If your sleep problems don't improve, consider seeking professional help to treat your insomnia and evaluate whether other sleep disorders, such as obstructive sleep apnea (in which breathing is interrupted several times during sleep) or periodic limb movement disorder, are playing a role.

An evaluation may involve a consultation with a sleep specialist (he/she should be certified by the American Academy of Sleep Medicine) and possibly an overnight sleep observation. A sleep center is usually the best place to receive such an evaluation. To find one, go to *www.sleepeducation.org/find-a-facility*. Insurance typically covers the cost.

To locate a therapist trained in CBT-I, consult the Association for Behavioral and Cognitive Therapies, *www.abct.org*. Four to eight sessions are typical, and in some cases, they are covered by insurance.

Sleep Your Way To Skinny

Michael Breus, PhD, is a clinical psychologist, diplomate of the American Board of Sleep Medicine and fellow of the American Academy of Sleep Medicine. He is the coauthor of *The Sleep Doctor's Diet Plan: Lose Weight Through Better Sleep.* Dr. Breus maintains a private practice in Scottsdale, Arizona. *TheSleep Doctor.com*

When we burn the midnight oil because we're just too busy for bed, it seems reasonable to expect that we would burn extra calories, too. But that's not what happens. In fact, the opposite is true. As a growing amount of research reveals, skimping on sleep is likely to make the number on the scale climb.

This seems unfair, especially when we're working so hard to stay slim (another celery stick, anyone?). But we might as well face facts if we hope to avoid getting fat. That's why I contacted Michael Breus, PhD, author of *The Sleep Doctor's Diet Plan: Lose Weight Through Better Sleep*, who explained the various factors that contribute to this connection.

Why sleep loss leads to weight gain…

• **Appetite-regulating hormones get out of balance.** Ghrelin is the "go" hormone that stimulates hunger…and when you're sleep-deprived, ghrelin levels increase by up to 15%, Dr. Breus said. Leptin is the "stop" hormone that tells you when you're full…and lack of sleep depletes leptin levels by about 20%, he added.

Curious finding: A study from St. Luke's/Roosevelt Hospital in New York City found that these hormonal effects differ by sex, with sleep-deprived women being particularly affected by the reduction in leptin and sleep-deprived men being particularly affected by the increase in ghrelin.

• **Your body goes into stress mode.** Loss of sleep leads to stress—and elevated levels of the stress hormone cortisol. This in turn is likely to trigger cravings, particularly for sugary or salty "comfort foods," such as cookies or chips.

• **Fat-cell activity goes awry.** A recent study from the University of Chicago found that when participants got 4.5 hours of sleep per night for four consecutive nights, their fat cells' response to insulin diminished by 30%. Dr. Breus explained that this decreases the ability of fat cells to properly store and release energy—so the body basically hangs onto calories rather than burning them.

• **Decision-making ability is compromised.** In a study from the University of California, Berkeley, MRI scans revealed that sleep-deprived people had significantly impaired activity in the frontal lobe of the brain, a region critical for making complex choices such as which foods to eat. As Dr. Breus explained it, a well-rested brain is more likely to make well-considered decisions, whereas a too-tired brain is prone to impulsiveness—including poor dietary decisions.

SLEEP-BOOSTING SCHEDULING SECRETS

Now that we've covered why sleep is so important for weight control, let's talk about how much sleep we need...and how to get it.

Though individual needs vary, research suggests that women with the healthiest weight-to-height ratio spend, on average, 7.7 hours in bed each night. If you're not coming close to that, take a look at your daily schedule. You could be sabotaging yourself with activities that interfere with your ability to fall asleep and stay asleep.

Here's how to adjust your routine...

• **Exercise early.** Regular physical activity promotes proper rest—but don't schedule your workout within four hours of bedtime or you may be too physically overstimulated to get to sleep.

• **Eat dinner three to four hours before bedtime.** When your stomach is too full, the sleep process has to compete with the digestive process, which can make it hard to get to sleep. But don't go to bed too hungry, either—hunger elevates cortisol levels, keeping you awake.

Dr. Breus's recommendations: If you need an after-dinner snack, have it at least an hour before bedtime...limit the snack to no more than 200 calories...and include a small amount of protein plus some complex carbohydrates. Good options include yogurt with almonds and granola...or warm oatmeal with milk and banana slices.

• **Avoid caffeine after 2 pm.** Caffeine can stay in your system for eight to 10 hours, so a late-afternoon latte could still be creating a sleep-stealing buzz past midnight.

• **Don't drink alcohol within three hours of bedtime.** Although a drink might help you fall asleep initially, alcohol reduces rapid eye movement (REM) sleep—so you won't feel well-rested come morning.

Better than a nightcap: Have some herbal tea sprinkled with nutmeg—the spice has been shown to promote slumber.

Trouble Falling Asleep? Stop Trying

Timothy I. Morgenthaler, MD, is a professor of medicine at The Center for Sleep Medicine at the Mayo Clinic in Rochester, Minnesota. He is the author of numerous medical journal articles on sleep and a member of the boards of directors of the American Academy of Sleep Medicine, the American Sleep Medicine Foundation and the American Board of Sleep Medicine.

If at first you don't succeed, try, try again? That's not good advice when it comes to dealing with insomnia, we hear from Mayo Clinic sleep expert Timothy I. Morgenthaler, MD, lead author of a guide to treating insomnia published in the journal *Sleep*. He explained that people who have trouble falling asleep or staying asleep often develop "performance anxiety"—so instead of relaxing and dropping off when they get into bed, they begin worrying, How long will it take me to fall asleep? Will I be able to stay asleep? The harder they try to drop off, the more tension that effort creates...and the tension keeps them from sleeping.

Solution: A technique called paradoxical intention is a kind of "reverse psychology" tool that anyone with any type of insomnia can use to break the performance anxiety cycle, Dr. Morgenthaler said. Basically, instead of trying to sleep, you try to not try to sleep. Known as a cognitive restructuring technique, this helps you stop dwelling on the problem. The idea isn't to force yourself to remain awake, but rather to get into bed, relax and shift your focus to positive, non-sleep-related thoughts. Recall the good things that happened during the day...indulge in a favorite relaxation technique, such as deep breathing or progressive muscle relaxation...enjoy your physical comfort...and appreciate how pleasant it is to be resting and not up working.

For people whose persistent insomnia has made them so anxious that even the thought of bed makes them physically keyed up, paradoxical intention may not work on the first try, Dr. Morgenthaler noted. If that is your situation and you feel yourself becoming frustrated, get up, leave the bedroom and do something passively relaxing that occupies your mind. Read, work a puzzle, knit or do whatever helps you unwind and shift gears mentally. Skip the TV and computer, however—it is best not to shine the bright light of a screen into your eyes, Dr. Morgenthaler said. When you are feeling drowsy, get back into bed and instead of thinking about sleep, simply focus on how good it feels to rest. This helps slumber come…effortlessly.

Surprising Solution For Restless Legs

Erez Salik, MD, is codirector of the Greenwich Vein Center in Greenwich, Connecticut, and a specialist in vascular and interventional radiology. *Greenvein.com*

You almost dread lying down because you know you'll soon feel that creepy-crawly, achy-tingly sensation in your legs. Moving your legs brings relief, so you can't resist the urge—but that makes it hard to fall asleep. The culprit is restless legs syndrome (RLS), a malady that affects about 10% of the population, with women being twice as prone to the problem as men. In many patients, RLS is primarily a neurological disorder. But in some, RLS has a different underlying cause that doctors often overlook—varicose veins.

Erez Salik, MD, codirector of the Greenwich Vein Center in Greenwich, Connecticut, explained that varicose veins develop when the one-way valves inside the leg veins, which are supposed to keep blood moving toward the heart, start to leak or fail. This allows blood to flow back toward the feet and pool in the legs. The increased pressure stretches the veins, causing them to become enlarged, twisted and bumpy. This inefficient circulation in the legs leads to a buildup of metabolic waste and can trigger the throbbing, itching, gotta-move-or-go-crazy sensations of RLS.

Good news: Treating the underlying vein problem also relieves RLS symptoms for many patients.

A simple, inexpensive, noninvasive treatment is to wear compression stockings (sold at drugstores and medical supply stores) because the stockings exert pressure that helps prevent the backflow and pooling of blood. Stockings are particularly helpful during long periods of standing but can be worn throughout the day and even at night, Dr. Salik said.

If compression stockings don't bring sufficient relief, consult an interventional radiologist, dermatologist or vascular surgeon with special training in phlebology (vein disorders). Referrals: Society of Interventional Radiology (*www. sirweb.org*)…or American College of Phlebology (*www.phlebology.org*). A physical exam and perhaps an ultrasound evaluation can help determine the most appropriate treatment.

Varicose veins often can be treated with minimally invasive procedures that are done in the doctor's office, involve minimal discomfort and take less than an hour, after which you walk out of the office. *Options may include…*

• **Endovenous laser ablation,** in which the doctor inserts a tiny tube into the vein, then heat energy from the device permanently seals the vein shut. This procedure is done using local anesthesia. In one study published in the journal *Phlebology*, patients who underwent this procedure experienced an average 80% improvement in their RLS symptoms…and 31% of participants got complete relief from RLS. *Average cost:* About $2,000 per leg.

• **Sclerotherapy,** in which the doctor injects the vein with a solution that causes the vein to scar, thus eventually closing the vein. No anesthesia is required. Some veins may need to be injected more than once in separate treatment sessions. *Average cost:* About $300 to $500 per session.

"With either treatment, the body automatically routes the blood to other, healthy veins, improving the circulation in the leg," Dr. Salik said. When varicose veins are treated strictly for cosmetic reasons, insurance generally does not pay. However, insurance often does cover the cost of treatment when a patient suffers from varicose vein–related symptoms, including RLS—a fact that should help you sleep better at night.

Natural Relief for Restless Legs

Chris D. Meletis, ND, executive director, Institute for Healthy Aging, Carson City, Nevada, a private practitioner in Beaverton, Oregon, and coauthor of *Great Health*.

I n bed, you feel an aching, tingling or "creepy-crawly" sensation in your legs. Moving brings relief, so you can't resist—but then it's hard to fall asleep.

Culprit: Restless legs syndrome (RLS), a neurological disorder that's twice as common in women as men. Sedative medications don't fully alleviate symptoms and can cause daytime drowsiness. *Better...*

●**Get screened for underlying conditions.** Diagnosis and treatment of diabetes, Parkinson's, sleep apnea or nerve damage may also relieve RLS.

●**Review medications.** Certain antihistamines, antidepressants, antinausea drugs and blood pressure drugs aggravate RLS. Ask your doctor about alternatives.

●**Take supplements.** Try this daily regimen for a month. If it helps, continue indefinitely—200 mg of alpha-lipoic acid...300 mg of magnesium...1,000 micrograms (mcg) of methyl-cobalamin, a form of vitamin B-12...800 mcg of 5-methyltetrahydrofolate (5-MTHF), a form of folic acid...and 300 mg of resveratrol. As with any supplement regimen, talk to your doctor before beginning.

●**Have your iron tested.** Iron deficiency increases RLS risk.

But: Excess iron can harm the brain and organs. Take iron only if a blood test reveals a deficiency and your doctor recommends it.

●**Use homeopathy.** Try Arsenicum album if RLS is accompanied by exhaustion and heaviness or trembling in the legs...Causticum if symptoms include burning or cramping in calves and feet...Ignatia if you have muscle spasms when dropping off to sleep. Consult a homeopathic practitioner for dosages.

●**Try acupuncture.** Some patients report improvement in RLS symptoms.

Symptom soother: Firmly massage your calves and thighs.

Don't Let Your Bed Partner Ruin Your Sleep—Simple Solutions for the Most Common Problems

Jeffry H. Larson, PhD, a licensed marriage and family therapist for more than 25 years and a professor of marriage and family therapy at the College of Family, Home and Social Sciences at Brigham Young University in Provo, Utah. He is the author of *Should We Stay Together? A Scientifically Proven Method for Evaluating Your Relationship and Improving Its Chances for Long-Term Success* and *The Great Marriage Tune-Up Book: A Proven Program for Evaluating and Renewing Your Relationship*, among other books. Dr. Larson also was the editor of the *Journal of Couple & Relationship Therapy.*

S ooner or later, one in every four American couples ends up sleeping in separate beds. Maybe it's your spouse's tossing and turning or TV watching in bed. Whatever the reason, it may seem easier just to turn that spare bedroom into a nighttime sanctuary of your own. But is that arrangement healthy?

New thinking: Even with the challenges that can come with sharing a bed, the net effect is usually positive for your health. While the exact mechanism is unknown, scientists believe that sleeping with a bed partner curbs levels of the stress hormone cortisol and inflammation-promoting proteins known as cytokines...while boosting levels of the so-called "love" hormone oxytocin.

Sleeping in the same bed also cultivates feelings of intimacy and security, which can strengthen a relationship and promote better sleep—factors linked to living a longer life. *Here, six common challenges and how to overcome them...*

●**You like to keep the room dark, while your partner prefers it light.** Sleep experts recommend keeping the room dark to help stimulate the production of the naturally occurring sleep hormone melatonin.

My advice: Room-darkening shades or light-blocking curtains help create the darkness we need for a good night's rest. But if your partner insists on having some light in the room, consider placing a dim night-light near his/her side of the bed. The person who prefers darkness may want to wear a sleep mask.

●**You're always cold, but your bed partner is too warm.** Sleep experts agree that a cooler room is generally more conducive to sleep and complements the natural temperature drop that occurs in the body when you go to sleep.

My advice: Optimal room temperature for the best sleep varies from person to person—most insomnia experts recommend a range of 60°F to 68°F. To help achieve your personal comfort level, use separate blankets so you can easily cover yourself or remove the blanket during the night without disturbing your bed partner. If you like to use an electric blanket during the winter, choose one with separate temperature controls.

●**You're a night owl, but your partner is a lark.** If the two bed partners prefer different bedtimes, this can cause both of them to lose sleep and can be a major contributor to marital strife. In a study involving 150 couples, which I conducted with several colleagues at Brigham Young University, the University of Nebraska–Lincoln and Montana State University, those who had mismatched body clocks argued more, spent less time doing shared activities and had slightly less sex.

The first step in trying to resolve conflicting bedtimes is to understand that one's circadian rhythm, the internal body clock that regulates sleep and wakefulness as well as other biological processes, dictates whether you are a natural early riser or a night owl. One's particular circadian rhythm is determined by genetics but can be influenced by sunlight, time zone changes and work schedules. Bedtime tendencies also can be socially learned.

My advice: Have a conversation with your partner. Avoid blaming the other party for having a different sleep schedule—we can't control our circadian rhythms or such factors as work schedules. Then, like everything else in a partnership, you'll need to compromise.

For instance, say your partner likes to go to bed at 10 pm and get up at 6 am, while you're rarely in bed before 1 am and sleep until 10 am. As a compromise, you might agree to get in bed with your partner at 9:30 pm to talk, snuggle, relax, read together, etc. Then, when your partner is ready to go to sleep, you can get up and continue with your night. Alternatively, you and your partner could agree to go to bed at the same time two or three nights a week. A night owl could also lie in bed and listen to music or an audiobook with headphones while his partner sleeps.

●**Your bed partner wants to watch TV, but you want peace and quiet.** Watching TV—or looking at any illuminated screen, such as a laptop or smartphone—promotes wakefulness and can interfere with sleep. So it's not really something anyone should do just before lights out. However, if one partner wants to watch TV or use a laptop before bed, he should do it in another room.

●**Your partner thrashes all night long.** Some individuals are naturally restless sleepers, tossing and turning throughout the night. Others may have restless legs syndrome (RLS) and/or periodic limb movement disorder (PLMD)—two related but distinct conditions.

RLS causes unpleasant sensations, such as tingling and burning, in the legs and an overwhelming urge to move them when the sufferer is sitting or attempting to sleep. PLMD causes involuntary movements and jerking of the limbs during sleep—the legs are most often affected but arm movements also can occur.

With RLS, the sufferer is aware of the problem. Individuals with PLMD, on the other hand, frequently are not aware that they move so much.

My advice: To help ease symptoms, you may want to try natural strategies such as taking warm baths, walking regularly and/or using magnesium supplements, which also promote sleep. But be sure to check with a doctor. If you have RLS or PLMD, it could signal an underlying health condition, such as iron deficiency.

If symptoms persist, you may want to talk to the doctor about medications such as *ropinirole* (Requip) and *pramipexole* (Mirapex), which can help relieve symptoms. Side effects may include nausea and drowsiness.

•**Your partner snores a lot—and loudly.** This is not only a nuisance, it also makes it hard for you to sleep.

My advice: In some cases, running a fan, listening to music through earbuds or using a white-noise machine can help.

If the snoring occurs almost every night, however, your partner may need to see an otolaryngologist (ear, nose and throat doctor) to determine whether there's an underlying medical condition.

Loud snoring that is accompanied by periods in which the person's breathing stops for a few seconds and then resumes may indicate sleep apnea, a serious—but treatable—disorder usually caused by a blocked or narrowed airway.

Trouble Sleeping? You May Be at Risk

Women who take longer than 30 minutes to fall asleep have a higher risk for diabetes, heart disease and stroke.

Reason: These women tend to have higher levels of insulin…inflammatory proteins that are linked to heart disease…and fibrinogen, a protein that is associated with stroke and heart attack.

Best: If you often have difficulty sleeping, talk to your doctor about the risks and ways to fall asleep.

Edward Suarez, PhD, professor, department of psychiatry and Behavioral Sciences, Duke University School of Medicine, Durham, North Carolina, and leader of a study of 210 people, published in *Brain, Behavior, and Immunity*.

Sleep Disorders Increase Risk for Depression

In a recent finding, men with sleep apnea—a condition characterized by snoring and interruptions in breathing while sleeping—were twice as likely to be depressed as men who did not have the condition. Women with sleep apnea were five times as likely to be depressed. Depression was most likely in people who had difficulties five or more nights a week.

Study of 9,714 men and women by researchers at the Centers for Disease Control and Prevention, Atlanta, published in *Sleep*.

Sleep Like a Baby

When 12 adult volunteers were asked to take a nap in an experimental hammock that either remained stationary or gently rocked, all of the participants who were rocked fell asleep faster and had more brain activity characteristic of restful sleep.

Current Biology

Better Way to Fall Asleep

Fifty-one adults who had difficulty falling asleep (sleep-onset insomnia) were divided into two groups. Both groups were taught good sleep practices (maintaining a standard wake-up time, using the bed only for sleeping, etc.). One group, however, also received cognitive refocusing therapy (CRT)—which involves thinking about something interesting but unexciting, such as song lyrics or recipes, when preparing for sleep or upon wakening during the night. After one month, the CRT group fell asleep much faster than the group that didn't do CRT. If you try CRT but insomnia persists, see a sleep medicine specialist.

Les A. Gellis, PhD, assistant clinical professor of practice psychology, College of Arts and Sciences, Syracuse University, New York.

Foods for Better Sleep...

Try salmon and spinach salad for dinner at 7 pm—omega-3s in the fish help you relax, and magnesium in spinach can calm your nerves. For dessert at 7:30, eat tart cherries—they contain the sleep hormone melatonin—or drink tart cherry juice. For a bedtime snack at 9 pm, make warm milk part of a soothing ritual—it is the routine, not the tryptophan in the milk, that is calming.

Health. Health.com

Sleeping With Your Partner Is Good for Your Health

Women in stable relationships who slept with their partners fell asleep faster and had fewer nighttime awakenings than women who slept alone.

Possible reason: Sleeping together lowers stress hormones and increases levels of oxytocin, the so-called love hormone, which reduces blood pressure.

Study of 35 married couples by researchers at University of Pittsburgh, quoted in *Health*.

Sleep Right to Fight Breast Sag

Do you usually sleep on your side? If you want to keep your breasts as perky as possible, you might want to rethink that habit. "Side-sleeping leaves the breasts hanging, so over time, it encourages them to sag," stated Christopher Rose, MD, medical director of the sleep labs at Covenant Health in Lubbock, Texas.

Sleeping on your stomach isn't smart, either. It squashes the breasts and promotes wrinkling—not to mention distorting the alignment of your neck and spine.

Best for breasts (and the rest of your body): Sleep on your back, Dr. Rose advised.

Exception: Pregnant women should avoid back-sleeping in the later months to keep the weight of the growing fetus off the intestines and major blood vessels (the aorta and vena cava), so that blood flows more freely to the fetus.

Christopher Rose, MD, is medical director of the sleep labs at Covenant Health in Lubbock, Texas.

8

Healthy Digestion

What to Eat to Beat Bloat

What's good for belly bloat? We contacted registered dietitians Lyssie Lakatos, RD, and Tammy Lakatos Shames, RD, who are twins and coauthors of *The Secret to Skinny: How Salt Makes You Fat and the 4-Week Plan to Drop a Size & Get Healthier with Simple Low-Sodium Swaps,* to find out which foods and beverages can help...and which to avoid.

Among the bloat-promoting culprits, first and foremost is salt. "Our bodies work to keep sodium levels at a certain balance. When we eat a lot of salt, our bodies respond by holding on to water to dilute the sodium and maintain it at the proper concentration. The bloat remains until you drink enough water to wash out the sodium—or until you eat foods that are high in both water and potassium. This mineral helps the body eliminate sodium via a mechanism called the sodium-potassium pump, whereby sodium is pumped out of cells and exchanged for potassium," Lakatos explained.

Potassium-rich antibloaters: Apricots, cantaloupe, citrus fruits, mangos, papayas and watermelon...and asparagus, beet greens, cucumbers, kale, spinach and tomatoes.

Constipation is another common contributor to bloating. When things are backed up, certain high-fiber foods come in especially handy. Lakatos and Shames call these particular fruits and vegetables flushers because they "flush you from the inside out" by creating a stool that can be easily eliminated—but without contributing as many calories as other high-fiber foods, such as whole grains.

Lyssie Lakatos, RD, LD, CDN, CFT, and Tammy Lakatos Shames, RD, LD, CDN, CFT, are the coauthors of *The Secret to Skinny: How Salt Makes You Fat and the 4-Week Plan to Drop a Size & Get Healthier with Simple Low-Sodium Swaps* and *Fire Up Your Metabolism.* The twins have appeared on numerous national television shows and are in private practice in New York City. *Nutrition Twins.com*

High-fiber flushers: Apples, berries, currants, figs, kiwifruit, oranges, pears, prunes and raisins…and bell peppers, broccoli, Brussels sprouts, cabbage, carrots, cauliflower, pumpkin and spaghetti squash.

You should get 14 grams of fiber per 1,000 calories—which works out to about 25 grams of fiber each day, or 21 grams if you're over 50 (because you need fewer calories when you're older).

But: If your body isn't used to that much fiber, it is best to increase your intake slowly. Otherwise, you may find yourself feeling more bloated thanks to gas. It also is important to drink enough water so all that fiber doesn't get stuck in your intestines, Shames said.

Rule of thumb: Drink two and a half to three ounces of water for every one gram of fiber.

Fruit quandary: Some people have a condition called fructose malabsorption, in which the body cannot properly absorb the fruit sugar fructose. After eating fruits that contain more fructose than glucose, they experience bloating and other gastrointestinal symptoms. Unfortunately, some fruits that serve as anti-bloaters or flushers for most folks—including apples, dried fruits, mangos, pears and watermelon—actually worsen bloating in these individuals. If you become more bloated after eating any of these foods, talk to your doctor about fructose malabsorption.

Surprising bloat promoters: Did you know that chewing gum and sipping through a straw (not necessarily at the same time!) can cause belly bloat by drawing excess air into your stomach? Carbonated beverages also leave your stomach full of gas.

The fix: Skip the gum and straws, and switch to nonsparkling drinks.

Watch out, too, for sugary foods. Lakatos told me that sugar works much the same way as sodium—when there's too much of it in your system, your body holds on to extra water to dilute it. So, instead of indulging in super-sugary desserts, try having a small handful of dried tart cherries or a few fresh dates or figs rolled in cocoa powder. These treats are sweet enough to satisfy your cravings but not so high in sugar that they'll leave you bloated.

Occasionally, bloating can be a sign of an underlying medical condition (such as irritable bowel syndrome, a pancreatic problem or colon cancer), so if puffiness persists, it is best to see your doctor. For most people, however, following the advice above will go a long way toward banishing bloat.

The Silent Cause of Stomach Trouble

Alessio Fasano, MD, chief, division of pediatric gastroenterology and nutrition at Massachusetts General Hospital in Boston, Massachusetts, where he is the director of the Center for Celiac Research & Treatment. He cochaired the international committee that published recent classifications for gluten-related disorders.

If you've always assumed that gluten-free foods are for someone else, it may be time to reconsider. Scientists are now finding that many more people than once believed are suffering ill effects from bread, cereal, pasta and other foods that contain gluten.

Until recently, most doctors thought that you could safely consume gluten unless you had celiac disease, an autoimmune disorder that damages the intestine and causes symptoms such as abdominal pain, bloating, chronic diarrhea and/or foggy thinking.

Now: An international panel of experts recently concluded that millions of Americans who do not have celiac disease also could benefit from giving up gluten. A new classification system, published in the peer-reviewed online journal *BMC Medicine* by BioMed Central, now identifies gluten sensitivity as a distinct disease, one that's related to, but not the same as, celiac disease.

It's an important distinction because people who tested negative for celiac disease in the past often were told that they didn't need to give up gluten, even when their symptoms were virtually identical to those of celiac patients. Some doctors even insisted that the symptoms were imaginary—and that these patients should get psychiatric help.

Gluten sensitivity also can lead to other conditions, such as irritable bowel syndrome (IBS), fibromyalgia and chronic fatigue syndrome.

We now know that gluten sensitivity is not only real but common, possibly affecting about 5% to 7% of Americans. Celiac disease affects about 1%. Could gluten be affecting you—and you don't even know it?

WHAT'S THE DIFFERENCE?

If you have celiac disease or gluten sensitivity, your immune system reacts to gluten—but in different ways…

With celiac disease, gluten triggers the activation of the immune system, which mistakenly attacks the small intestine. A similar process is involved in other autoimmune diseases, such as rheumatoid arthritis and lupus.

If you have celiac disease and eat gluten, the immune system attacks villi, hairlike projections in the small intestine that absorb nutrients. Abdominal discomfort and digestive problems, including the malabsorption of essential vitamins and minerals, can result.

The symptoms can differ among celiac patients—some may have sharp abdominal pains that come and go…others could experience a chronic squeezing ache. They also can have a higher risk of developing intestinal cancer or neurological disorders, such as migraines and peripheral neuropathy.

With gluten sensitivity, a part of the immune system known as the innate immune system is affected. Unlike people with celiac disease, those with gluten sensitivity don't produce antibodies to gluten, nor do they suffer damage to the small intestine or have a higher-than-average risk for cancer. They do have an immediate reaction to gluten—the body releases inflammatory substances that can cause abdominal pain and other symptoms similar to those seen in celiac disease.

Similarly, a person who has a wheat allergy can have many of the same symptoms of celiac disease or gluten sensitivity. With a wheat allergy, however, the patient may have an itchy skin rash, asthma or even, in extreme cases, anaphylaxis, a severe, whole-body allergic reaction that can be life-threatening.

A GROWING THREAT

The incidence of celiac disease has quadrupled in about the last half-century. Researchers suspect that gluten sensitivity has increased at a similar rate. The reasons for these increases aren't yet known.

One possible explanation is that our bodies haven't had time to adapt to the processed foods and the increased gluten content found in several grains during the last 50 years. As a result, the immune systems in people genetically predisposed to gluten-related disorders may not recognize these foods as "friendly."

WHEN TO SUSPECT GLUTEN

Many people with celiac disease or gluten sensitivity eventually see a diet-related pattern to their symptoms—they feel worse when they eat such foods as bread and pasta.

Good news: The symptoms of both celiac disease and gluten sensitivity typically disappear following the adoption of a gluten-free diet. With celiac disease, symptoms may improve within a few weeks, although the intestinal damage may take several months or even years to completely heal. If you're sensitive to gluten, the relief can be much faster, often within a few days.

WHAT TESTS DO YOU NEED?

If you suspect that you have celiac disease, get tested before giving up gluten-containing foods. People with celiac disease who quit consuming gluten will have a false-negative blood test—it will show that they don't have the disease even if they really do. *Here's how celiac disease is detected…*

• **Blood test.** This is a simple and an accurate way to identify two antibodies, anti-endomysium and anti-tissue transglutaminase, that are produced when patients are exposed to gluten.

• **Biopsy.** A diagnosis of celiac disease (but not gluten sensitivity or a wheat allergy) can be verified with a biopsy. It's done by endoscopy, which involves the insertion of a thin tube through the mouth, esophagus and stomach and into the small intestine. A small piece of tissue is removed and examined in a laboratory to look for damage to the villi. Those with gluten sensitivity or wheat allergies will not have damaged villi.

There are no reliable tests for gluten sensitivity. The condition is a diagnosis of exclusion—your doctor will say that you have gluten sensitivity if you test negative for celiac disease and a wheat allergy (diagnosed by a skin prick or blood test), but your symptoms and personal history indicate gluten is the problem.

GO GLUTEN-FREE

If you have celiac disease, you must avoid all obvious and hidden sources of gluten for life. Widely recognized sources of gluten are wheat, barley and rye, and lesser-known sources include bulgar and spelt (both forms of wheat).

Ask your doctor for a referral to a licensed dietitian to help you adhere to the gluten-free diet. Read food labels to learn which packaged foods contain gluten, and join a support group in your area to learn about gluten-free resources. For a list of gluten-free foods, go to *www.Celiac.org*…or to get recipes, go to *www. Gluten.org*.

If you have gluten sensitivity, you also may need to follow a gluten-free diet. However, some people with gluten sensitivity can tolerate small amounts of gluten, such as a few bites of pizza or a taste of bread. In some cases, tolerance can change over time.

Caution: If you have celiac disease, even trace amounts of gluten can trigger a reaction. For example, foods without gluten, such as oats, can cause a problem for celiac sufferers if gluten-containing foods are processed on the same machinery.

WHAT IS GLUTEN?

Gluten is a protein that occurs naturally in wheat, barley and rye—as well as in bulgar and spelt (forms of wheat). Breads, cereals, pastas and cakes are among the foods that typically contain gluten. It also can be found in thousands of processed foods, including salad dressings, ice cream, yogurt and soup (often listed as "filler flour," "vegetable starch" and "hydrolyzed wheat gluten").

Postmenopausal Heartburn

Leo Galland, MD, director, Foundation for Integrated Medicine, New York City. He is author of *The Fat Resistance Diet. www.mdheal.org*. Dr. Galland is a recipient of the Linus Pauling Award.

D oes hormone replacement therapy cause heartburn? That was the implication of reports associating the heartburn suffered by many postmenopausal women with use of either over-the-counter estrogen (phytoestrogens/botanicals) or HRT. The data was from the Nurses' Health Study, which has been gathering information from more than 121,000 registered nurses since the 1970s.

Published in the *Archives of Internal Medicine*, the study reported that women who were using OTC products that are estrogen-based or who were on hormone replacement therapy were one-and-a-half times more likely to report having symptoms of heartburn or other gastroesophageal reflux disease (GERD) symptoms. Leo Galland, MD, director of the Foundation for Integrated Medicine, and author of the downloadable e-book *The Heartburn and Indigestion Solution*, believes the heartburn connection is more complex.

HORMONES AND GERD

The study associates the use of estrogen products with GERD (defined in the study as heartburn that occurs one or more times a week). However as we know, a correlation isn't the same as causation. Dr. Galland said that many factors may account for the increased risk of heartburn associated with hormone therapy used during or after menopause. Hormones like estrogen and progesterone affect how well muscles are able to contract, and therefore may contribute to heartburn by relaxing the LES valve that separates the stomach from the esophagus. This relaxation of the smooth muscle tissue in the lower esophagus lets stomach acid back up—that's what causes the burning sensation, Dr. Galland explained. It's thought that the presence of extra progesterone is probably responsible for heartburn that occurs during pregnancy and it's also a component in many treatments for menopausal symptoms.

It's important to take these and all GERD symptoms seriously, as left untreated, it can lead to precancerous tissue changes. "Prevention is important," says Dr. Galland. Taking calcium supplements is among the most effective ways to prevent GERD, he noted. He recommends following meals immediately with either a chewable product (like Viactiv or a drug store brand) or powdered calcium citrate that you dissolve in water and drink (several brands are available online). "These increase the tightness of the LES valve and also improve the ability of the esophagus to expel stomach acid back into the stomach," he explained.

In the meantime, if you experience heartburn, consider the possibility that hormones, drugs or dietary supplements you're taking may contribute to the symptoms and understand that these symptoms are likely not due to excess stomach acid, but to weakness of the LES valve. See a doctor for proper hormonal assessment and symptomatic management.

Drug-Free Help for Chronic Heartburn

Kristina Conner, ND, is an associate professor, clinical sciences, at National University of Health Sciences in Lombard, Illinois. She specializes in natural family medicine for women and children, naturopathic endocrinology and gastroenterology.

An estimated 20% of Americans have a chronic form of heartburn—characterized by chest pain, a persistent cough and/or burning at the back of the throat that occur more than twice weekly—known as gastroesophageal reflux disease (GERD). Besides causing significant discomfort, if left untreated, this condition increases the risk for esophageal cancer.

So it was unwelcome news when a recent article in the *Canadian Medical Association Journal* confirmed that two types of stomach-acid-reducing drugs commonly used to treat GERD are linked to increased risk for pneu-

monia. Long-term use of these drugs—proton pump inhibitors (such as Prilosec and Prevacid) and H-2 blockers (such as Tagamet and Zantac)—also is linked to impaired nutrient absorption...increased risk for hip fractures, high blood pressure and heart attack...and perhaps reduced effectiveness of the blood thinner *clopidogrel* (Plavix).

Fortunately: Drugs are not the only way to deal with GERD. Kristina Conner, ND, an associate professor, clinical sciences, at National University of Health Sciences in Lombard, Illinois, who specializes in women's health and digestive problems, told me about various natural therapies that ease or eliminate GERD.

A quick review of digestive biology...To break down food, the stomach produces about one quart of hydrochloric acid daily. At the base of the esophagus is the lower esophageal sphincter (LES), a band of muscle that opens to let swallowed food into the stomach, then shuts again. When the LES fails to close properly, stomach acid backs up into the esophagus and damages the esophageal lining. This is what happens with GERD. *What helps...*

ESOPHAGUS-SOOTHING SUPPLEMENTS

Taken alone or in combination for two to four months, the dietary supplements below promote esophageal healing, Dr. Conner said. For dosages and guidelines on which supplements are most appropriate for you, consult a naturopathic physician. *Options...*

• **Calcium citrate powder mixed with water** helps tighten the LES and improves the esophagus's ability to push acid back into the stomach.

• **Deglycyrrhized licorice tablets** promote production of mucus that protects esophageal cells.

• **Marshmallow root lozenges** contain mucilage, a gelatinous substance that coats the gastrointestinal tract, soothes inflammation and heals cells lining the esophagus and stomach, Dr. Conner said.

• **Slippery elm herbal tea** also provides mucilage. Drink it hot, not iced. Warm beverages are easier to absorb than cold drinks, which can tax gastrointestinal function, Dr. Conner pointed out.

Vitamin B complex, including thiamine (B-1), pantothenic acid (B-5) and choline, promotes proper smooth-muscle activity of the esophagus to keep food moving in the right direction.

ANTI-GERD DIET

Foods that can exacerbate GERD by relaxing the LES muscle and/or increasing acidity generally are those that are spicy or high in fat or sugar. Some people find that symptoms are triggered by certain other foods, such as alcohol, carbonated beverages, citrus fruits and juices, chocolate, coffee, mint, onions and tomatoes. Contrary to the popular idea that dairy foods ease GERD, they actually can worsen symptoms. "You do not necessarily need to give up all these foods forever, but you will feel better if you avoid them long enough to let your body recover," Dr. Conner said.

What to do: Eliminate all potential troublemakers from your diet for two to four weeks, then reintroduce them one at a time. If eating a particular food brings on symptoms within a day, avoid it for another three to six months, then try it again. If GERD symptoms return, it is best to avoid this food henceforth. If no symptoms develop after the three- to six-month hiatus, you may be able to eat this food occasionally. But keep portions moderate. "You can't drink eight cups of coffee or soda per day and expect GERD not to return," Dr. Conner noted.

Safe to eat: Foods unlikely to exacerbate GERD include those that are high in fiber, complex carbohydrates and/or minerals, Dr. Conner said. Good choices include most fruits and vegetables (except those identified above as potential heartburn triggers)…lean meats and skinless poultry…and whole grains.

Eat slowly and chew carefully, giving your mouth—a key part of your digestive system—and stomach plenty of time to work. Don't overfill your stomach. "Avoid eating while watching TV, driving, standing up or doing anything that takes attention away from your food and encourages you to rush or overeat," Dr. Conner said.

Celebrate your food: Put out placemats, cloth napkins, even candles…as you eat, notice each food's taste, texture and aroma. You'll enjoy your food more and eat less—a double benefit.

Relief from IBS Naturally

Andrew L. Rubman, ND, medical director, Southbury Clinic for Traditional Medicines, Southbury, Connecticut. *SouthburyClinic.com*

Sometimes old-fashioned remedies work best, and for the millions of people with one very hard-to-treat condition—irritable bowel syndrome (IBS)—an old remedy beats everything modern science has dreamed up. If you or someone you know has IBS, please read on.

As many as one in five Americans suffer from IBS, a miserable disorder that can bring an endless progression of constipation, diarrhea, gas, bloating and stomach cramps. Where expensive new IBS drugs have been disappointing, it turns out that a classic stomachache remedy, peppermint oil, can often get the job done more effectively.

IN WITH THE OLD, OUT WITH THE NEW

At McMaster University in Ontario, Alexander C. Ford, MD, and his colleagues analyzed the results of many previously published studies on adults with IBS, including 12 comparing fiber with placebo, 22 comparing antispasmodics with placebo, and four comparing peppermint oil with placebo. Peppermint oil was surprisingly effective, bringing relief to 74% of patients. This compares very favorably with antispasmodics, which helped only 61%, and fiber, which was beneficial to just 48%.

Peppermint oil may be most helpful in soothing the abdominal pain and cramping that are common IBS symptoms and, over time, it may also help ease diarrhea or constipation. Scientists believe it works by blocking the movement of calcium into muscle cells in the gastrointestinal tract, thereby reducing muscle contractions, discomfort and bloating.

HOW TO MAKE YOUR IBS BETTER

Look for "enteric coated" peppermint oil capsules at your health food store, since taking peppermint oil straight can produce reflux symptoms, suggests *Health Insider* contributing medical editor Andrew L. Rubman, ND. Dr. Rubman often prescribes doses of 200 mg to 300 mg to be taken once, twice or three times daily—but not more often, as larger doses can be toxic. He says most patients find it helpful to take a dose just before eating a meal.

Several factors should be weighed in identifying the right treatment for an IBS patient, including whether symptoms are dominated by diarrhea or constipation or whether both occur about equally. If your doctor seems quick to recommend newer pharmaceuticals, consider seeing a specialist in natural medicine to discuss the older remedies and over-the-counter medicines. Dr. Ford pointed out that even though peppermint oil helped the most people in his analysis, the other two treatments—fiber and antispasmodics (which lessen spasms in the GI tract)—were effective for many, and they are safe, inexpensive and readily available over the counter at most pharmacies. Also, Dr. Rubman said that there are many other useful botanical extracts that are antispasmodic as well, including valerian, skullcap, viburnum, juniper berry, hyoscamus niger, gentian and gelsemium. "Their effects may vary from minor to profound, so it's best to use these only under physician care," he added.

Hypnotherapy Eases Irritable Bowel Syndrome (IBS)

Scientists recently conducted research involving a total of 346 irritable bowel syndrome (IBS) patients to test the effectiveness of hypnotherapy as a treatment.

Result: Symptoms were satisfactorily reduced for 40% of patients who received one hour of hypnotherapy once a week for 12 weeks. The positive effect lasted for one to seven years.

Theory: IBS patients can learn to control their symptoms through deep relaxation and hypnotic suggestion.

Magnus Simrén, MD, PhD, professor of gastroenterology, The Sahlgrenska Academy's Institute of Medicine, University of Gothenburg, Sweden.

The Right Probiotic Can Relieve Digestive Complaints, Rheumatoid Arthritis and More

Gary B. Huffnagle, PhD, professor of internal medicine at the University of Michigan Medical School in Ann Arbor and coauthor of *The Probiotics Revolution: The Definitive Guide to Safe, Natural Health Solutions Using Probiotic and Prebiotic Foods and Supplements.*

Until recently, probiotics were mostly known for their ability to help prevent or alleviate various digestive problems.

Now: Research has uncovered several other health benefits—for example, these beneficial intestinal microorganisms also boost immunity and reduce the severity of certain autoimmune conditions, such as rheumatoid arthritis and asthma.

What you need to know...

THE RIGHT PROBIOTIC

Consuming probiotics is one of the smartest things you can do for your health.

What you may not know: Some probiotics—available as over-the-counter (OTC) supplements and in certain fermented food products, such as many brands of yogurt and buttermilk—have been found to be more effective than others for treating certain conditions.

What's more, because everyone's intestinal microflora—the term for the many billions of different bacteria and fungi that populate your gut—is unique in its exact makeup, a probiotic that's effective for someone else might not work for you, and vice versa.

Best approach: Try one probiotic product (such as those described in this article) for two weeks and see if you feel better. Probiotics are extremely safe. While some people may experience slight gastrointestinal disturbance, such as intestinal gas or bloating, from a given probiotic, this can be alleviated by reducing the dosage.

If you don't see clear benefits after two weeks, try a different probiotic from the same category.

Even though most research has focused on the benefits of single types (strains) of micro-organisms, many people benefit from combining two or more probiotics, and a number of probiotic products also contain multiple strains.

Once you find a probiotic you respond well to, I recommend taking it daily even in the absence of any specific health complaint—just like a daily multivitamin and mineral supplement.

Choose products from well-known manufacturers, such as Culturelle and Align, that include information on the label about the type of micro-organisms and number of viable bacteria, or colony-forming units (CFUs), they contain. Follow the label recommendation on dosage. Studies indicate that probiotics are equally effective when taken with or without food.

FOR DIGESTIVE PROBLEMS

In addition to promoting the growth of beneficial bacteria in the gut, probiotics aid digestion by inhibiting the proliferation of harmful bacteria and other micro-organisms in the intestines.

If you suffer from digestive problems, including diarrhea, constipation, bloating, gastroesophageal reflux disease or irritable bowel syndrome (IBS), try one of the following OTC probiotics…

•**Bifidobacterium.** This group, one of the major types of intestinal bacteria, includes Bifidobacterium infantis (found in Align, sold in capsule form)…Bifidobacterium bifidus (a common ingredient of many probiotic supplements, such as those by Source Naturals and Nature's Way)…and Bifidobacterium animalis (contained in Activia yogurt).

Important scientific evidence: In a 2006 randomized study of 362 women with IBS,

those who took B. infantis in a daily dose of 10 million CFUs showed significant improvement after four weeks, compared with a placebo group.

•**Bacillus coagulans.** This species of bacteria can survive for an extended time in the digestive tract, which is believed to increase the probiotic's effectiveness. In a 2009 study of 44 people with IBS, those receiving a daily dose of B. coagulans reported significant improvement.

FOR ALLERGIES, ASTHMA, ARTHRITIS, ECZEMA AND MORE

As a first-line probiotic for allergies, asthma, eczema or other autoimmune-related disorders, I recommend trying either B. coagulans—shown in a 2010 study to significantly reduce rheumatoid arthritis pain compared with a placebo—or one of the following…

•**Lactobacillus.** Another major category of probiotics, this genus includes the widely used Lactobacillus acidophilus, contained in many probiotic supplements and yogurt products (including Brown Cow, Stonyfield Farm and some Dannon yogurts)…Lacto-bacillus GG (the active ingredient in Culturelle capsules and powder)…and Lactobacillus casei (contained in the yogurt drink DanActive).

•**Saccharomyces boulardii.** This probiotic is actually a strain of yeast. Although most people think of yeast as something to be avoided—as in a yeast infection, for example—S. boulardii helps fight disease-causing organisms. S. boulardii is available in capsule form in Florastor and in products by Jarrow Formulas, NutriCology, Swanson, NOW Foods, Douglas Laboratories and others.

FOR COLDS AND FLU

While it is important that your immune system be activated to attack a cold or flu virus, many of the symptoms that make you feel sick from these ailments are actually side effects that occur due to the fact that your immune system is overreacting.

Probiotics can help you reduce symptoms, such as body aches, of colds or the flu. If you feel a cold or some other virus coming on, consider trying a Lactobacillus, B. coagulans or S. boulardii probiotic.

Some research suggests that probiotics also may help prevent urinary tract infections.

DURING ANTIBIOTIC TREATMENT

If you are taking a course of antibiotics, it is essential that you also take probiotics to help prevent adverse effects, such as diarrhea and yeast infection.

Reason: Antibiotics kill both infection-causing bacteria and beneficial bacteria. Probiotics will help restore these good bacteria. Any one of the probiotics listed earlier—including yogurt products—can be used.

It's important to start taking daily probiotics immediately after you've completed your antibiotic regimen and continue taking them for a few weeks.

You can also begin taking probiotics while you're on an antibiotic if desired. Just be sure to take the antibiotic four to six hours away from the probiotic to make sure the antibiotic is fully absorbed. This ensures that the probiotic will not interfere with the antibiotic's ability to fight infection.

PROBIOTIC-BOOSTING DIET

Certain foods, known as "prebiotics," stay in the digestive tract for an extended period of time, where they stimulate the growth of many types of beneficial bacteria.

Try to include as many of the following prebiotic foods in your diet as possible each day. For example...

Foods rich in natural anti-oxidants—especially those found in colorful fruits and vegetables, such as berries, citrus fruits, peppers, tomatoes, broccoli, spinach, asparagus and okra...dark beans and nuts...and green tea.

Foods high in soluble fiber—including legumes, such as peas, lentils and pinto beans...oat bran...carrots and Brussels sprouts...apples, pears and prunes...and root vegetables, such as onions and unprocessed potatoes.

To further boost soluble fiber consumption: Talk to your doctor about taking a daily psyllium supplement, such as Carlson Psyllium Fiber Supplement or Metamucil. Follow label instructions.

At the same time, minimize your intake of processed foods containing sugar, white flour and other refined carbohydrates—all of which promote the growth of harmful bacteria in the digestive tract.

Surprising Foods That Can Upset Your Stomach

Christine L. Frissora, MD, assistant attending physician at New York-Presbyterian Hospital and an associate professor of medicine at Weill Medical College of Cornell University, both in New York City.

If you have a sensitive stomach, you probably experience frequent bouts of digestive distress. While in some cases it's obvious what has caused the discomfort—for example, eating spicy foods or taking seconds, or even thirds—other times it seems to be a mystery.

What you may not know is that it could have been something seemingly harmless, or even healthful—like green tea or yogurt—that caused you to feel nauseated or bloated.

FOODS TO AVOID

Surprising triggers of digestive discomfort...

• **Energy bars.** Because these bars, such as ZonePerfect bars and PowerBars, contain added nutrients and vitamins, they typically are eaten as a healthful snack, a meal replacement or for a preworkout energy boost. Some bars, especially low-sugar or low-carb varieties, contain sugar alcohols, such as glycerin and maltitol syrup, which can cause bloating, gas and diarrhea. Other bars are simply too high in complex carbohydrates and calories for someone with a sensitive stomach to digest easily.

What to do: If you want to have an energy bar, be sure to eat only a small portion of it at a time.

• **Green tea.** Although green tea is widely recognized for its disease-fighting properties—it's full of antioxidants and other compounds that help fight cancer and heart disease and stave off diabetes, stroke and dementia—it contains irritants that can make you feel nauseated.

For example, green tea contains caffeine—anywhere from 24 mg to 40 mg per eight-ounce cup—which can irritate the gastrointestinal (GI) tract. Even decaffeinated green tea has some caffeine. But it's not the caffeine by itself that makes green tea a cause of digestive distress in some people. Green tea is also very high in tannins (polyphenols responsible for its astringent taste), which are associated with nausea and stomach upset in some individuals.

What to do: If green tea makes you nauseated, avoid it altogether or have a very weak cup. Chamomile tea is soothing to the GI tract and is a good alternative.

•**Vegetable skins.** Eggplant, bell pepper and potato skins can be difficult to digest, especially if you have diverticulitis (inflamed or infected pouches in the intestinal wall) or colitis (inflammation of the large intestine)… or have had complicated abdominal surgery (involving infection or perforation).

What to do: Peel thick-skinned vegetables, then purée, mash or stew the insides before eating to aid digestion.

•**Grapes.** Red and black grapes contain the phytochemical resveratrol, a powerful antioxidant thought to help protect against coronary disease, some cancers and viral infections. But eating too many grapes—or even just a few if you are sensitive to them—can cause nausea and diarrhea. *Reason:* Grapes are high in fructose, a natural sugar that often causes gas. Green grapes contain a lot of tannins, like green tea, which can lead to stomach upset.

What to do: Eat only a small amount of grapes, or avoid them altogether if you are sensitive to them. Instead, try eating other fruits rich in resveratrol, such as cranberries, blueberries and bilberries.

•**Nuts.** The high fiber and fat content of nuts slow their movement through the digestive tract, which increases the risk for gas and bloating. Nuts also contain stomach-irritating tannins.

What to do: Avoid eating nuts if you experience digestive discomfort when consuming them…have had a complicated abdominal

surgery…have peritonitis (inflammation of the inner abdominal wall)…or have diverticulosis (small pouches that bulge through the large intestine) or diverticulitis. Some alternatives to whole nuts include nut butters or oatmeal with berries.

•**Probiotics.** The balance of healthful and potentially unhealthful bacteria in your digestive system can be thrown off due to illness, medications and diet, causing diarrhea and constipation. Probiotic supplements and foods contain live, healthful bacteria that can help restore balance to the digestive system. Examples of the bacteria contained in probiotics include Lactobacillus and Bifidobacterium.

Certain probiotic supplements and foods are helpful for specific situations. For example, Activia yogurt can help alleviate constipation… the supplement Align can ease bloating…and Florastor (Saccharomyces boulardii lyo) helps diarrhea caused by antibiotics.

What to do: Many probiotic supplements and foods can produce bloating (due to the ingestion of billions of bacteria). Avoid probiotics if this is a problem for you.

Caution: If you are severely ill or your immune system is compromised, avoid probiotics (and check with your doctor before having yogurt). Probiotics can enter the bloodstream and cause sepsis, a potentially life-threatening condition caused by the body's inflammatory response to bacteria or other germs.

Important: A sensitive stomach, marked by gas and bloating, may be caused by celiac disease, an immune reaction to gluten in wheat, barley and rye. If you have these symptoms, get tested for celiac disease.

BETTER-KNOWN TROUBLEMAKERS

You may already know that the following foods can cause stomach upset, but they're worth a reminder…

•**Artificial sweeteners.** Some artificial sweeteners, such as Splenda (sucralose), Equal (aspartame) and Sweet'N Low (saccharin), are difficult for the body to break down, which can lead to bloating, nausea, headache and other symptoms.

What to do: Be on the lookout for artificial sweeteners, which are found not only in diet sodas and sugarless gum, but also in many other processed foods, including some yogurts, cereals, snacks and juices.

• **Carbonated beverages.** These drinks contain carbon dioxide gas, which distends the stomach.

What to do: Avoid beer, soda, seltzer and other "fizzy" drinks if you have bloating. Plain water is best.

• **Monosodium glutamate (MSG).** This flavor enhancer often is added to Chinese food, canned vegetables, soups and processed meats. It can cause nausea, headache, cramping, fatigue and other symptoms.

What to do: Avoid Chinese food, unless it is free of MSG, and avoid canned or processed foods with MSG on the label.

WHAT HELPS

How you eat and drink also can help prevent discomfort. For example, it's widely known that having six small meals per day, rather than three larger meals, makes it easier for the stomach to empty properly. *Other helpful approaches...*

• **Drink liquids between meals.** While the digestive system needs to be well-hydrated to function optimally, too much water or other liquids during meals can overdistend the stomach, especially in patients with gastroesophageal reflux disease (GERD), in which stomach contents backwash into the esophagus...hiatal hernia, in which part of the stomach sticks upward into the chest through an opening in the diaphragm...and gastroparesis, delayed emptying of the stomach.

Small sips of liquid during a meal are fine.

Helpful: Avoid having a lot of liquids about 15 minutes before you eat and at least an hour after you eat.

• **Don't talk while eating.** This can lead to aerophagia, a condition caused by swallowing too much air, which can result in abdominal bloating, frequent belching and gas.

• **Eat slowly and chew well.** Make sure to thoroughly chew foods before swallowing.

• **Stew meats.** They are digested more easily than those that are broiled, grilled or fried.

• **Take chewable supplements.** Many supplements can cause bloating or nausea. If possible, use chewable forms, which are less likely to cause discomfort.

WHAT CAUSES A SENSITIVE STOMACH?

Your stomach mixes food with digestive juices, then empties its contents into the small intestine. If you have a sensitive stomach, the muscles of the stomach may function more slowly, which can lead to indigestion. Or the nerves of the stomach may be overly sensitive to distension (enlargement of the stomach after eating), resulting in uncomfortable bloating. Eating certain foods can make these symptoms worse.

The 10 Riskiest Foods for Food Poisoning

Barbara Kowalcyk, PhD, is cofounder and Board Director of the Center for Foodborne Illness Research & Prevention, a national nonprofit organization based in Raleigh, North Carolina. *FoodborneIllness.org*

"Foodborne illnesses are much more common than people think," says Barbara Kowalcyk, PhD, cofounder and Board Director of the Center for Foodborne Illness Research & Prevention. Indeed, according to the Centers for Disease Control and Prevention, one out of every six Americans, or 48 million people, are affected by foodborne illnesses each year...128,000 of them are hospitalized...and 3,000 die.

When your stomach is upset, how can you tell whether food poisoning is the culprit? You can't necessarily count on your last meal to give you a clue because incubation periods vary widely—from mere hours to weeks—depending on the specific pathogen causing the illness. Instead, consider the symptoms. "If you have diarrhea and vomiting, there's a good chance that you have a foodborne illness. Often people say, 'I have the stomach flu,' but there is no such thing—the flu is an upper respiratory infection, not a gastrointestinal problem," Dr. Kowalcyk said.

Which foods are riskiest? The answer depends on whom you ask. According to research from the University of Florida Emerging Pathogens Institute, the foods most likely to cause problems are poultry...nonmeat multi-ingredient dishes (such as sandwiches, sauces and pasta dishes)...pork...produce...beef...deli meats...dairy foods...seafood...game...eggs...baked goods...and beverages. But the Center for Science in the Public Interest (CSPI) says that the 10 riskiest foods among those regulated by the FDA are, in order, leafy greens...eggs...tuna...oysters...potatoes...cheese...ice cream...tomatoes...sprouts...and berries. (For info on why these particular foods comprise the top culprits, see the CSPI report at *http:// bit.ly/tQdzt.*)

The pathogens: There are two main types of pathogens that cause foodborne illnesses. *They are...*

•**Norovirus.** This is the most common and tends to peak in the colder months. It doesn't grow on food, but you can get it from food or drink that has been contaminated by coming in contact with the virus—from someone's unwashed hands, for instance, or from sharing utensils with an infected person. Primary symptoms include nausea, stomach cramps, vomiting and diarrhea...some infected people also experience fever, headaches and body aches. Because a patient might vomit or have diarrhea many times in one day, dehydration is a common side effect.

•**Bacteria.** Among those that cause food poisoning are Salmonella, Clostridium botulinum, Listeria monocytogenes and certain strains of Escherichia coli (E. coli), particularly O157:H7. These bacteria grow on the food itself. Summer is prime time for outbreaks because bacteria grow faster in warmer temperatures...and because at this time of year, people tend to eat more produce raw (cooking kills the bacteria). Symptoms are similar to those of norovirus but sometimes can be more dangerous. E. coli, for example, is linked to hemolytic-uremic syndrome (HUS), a disorder that can lead to kidney failure and death.

If you develop symptoms: Fortunately, most cases of food poisoning are relatively mild and symptoms usually subside on their own within a few days. During that time, it helps to stay hydrated by drinking over-the-counter oral rehydration fluids. However, you should see your doctor immediately if you experience any of the following...

•**Severe vomiting.**

•**Severe diarrhea...**any bloody diarrhea...or diarrhea that lasts more than a few days.

•**Symptoms that suggest severe dehydration** (scant or amber-colored urine, very dry mouth, skin that "tents" when pinched, sunken eyes, rapid heartbeat).

Testing determines the specific pathogen, which will dictate treatment. Dr. Kowalcyk said, "Without taking a stool sample and testing it, the doctor is not necessarily going to know the best way to treat you. For example, E. coli should not be treated with antibiotics, whereas some strains of Salmonella should be treated with antibiotics."

Whether or not you wind up needing a doctor, Dr. Kowalcyk recommended calling your county or state health department to report any suspected case of foodborne illness.

Reason: If you are at the beginning of an outbreak, alerting the authorities could help prevent more cases from developing—which means that your quick action potentially could save lives.

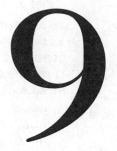

9

I Hate to Exercise And Diet

Have a Love Affair With Exercise...

Some people just seem to adore exercise. You see them at the gym or jogging around the neighborhood—sweating, smiling, looking fit. But if you would rather dive into a cauldron of boiling oil than work out on a regular basis, you probably wonder how other people can possibly enjoy exercise...and wish that you could, too.

Fact: You can learn to love exercise. Several simple behavioral changes can, within seven weeks, result in a major shift in the way you feel about physical activity.

WEEK ONE...

•**First, do nothing.** The number-one obstacle to exercise is lack of time. To overcome this, commit to a one-week predecision phase. You don't actually exercise yet—the purpose is to prove that your schedule can accommodate three 30-minute chunks of workout time

per week. How? Wake up a half-hour earlier than usual on, say, Tuesday, Thursday and Saturday...or take 30 minutes after work on Monday, Wednesday and Friday. During these times, do not make phone calls, check e-mail, pay bills or pick up clutter. Instead, just relax and imagine yourself doing different kinds of physical activities. *While you daydream...*

•**Open your mind.** Maybe you learned to hate exercise in your junior high school gym class when you were chosen last for a volleyball game or puffed around the track in an ill-fitting gym suit. That's understandable—but you don't have to let past unpleasantness poison your possibilities now. Instead, try to remember what you did enjoy as a youngster, such as riding a bike, jumping rope or playing softball. Or imagine doing something entirely new to you—for instance, a tai chi class or a Nintendo Wii Fit exercise video game. Notice how the thought of each option makes you

---

Mark Stibich, PhD, adjunct faculty member at the University of California, San Diego School of Medicine and expert on behavioral science.

feel. When an imagined activity gets you excited, write it down on a list.

WEEKS TWO AND THREE...

•**Start moving.** For the next two weeks, continue carving out your thrice-weekly half-hour periods, but instead of just visualizing exercise, do a little. Don't push yourself too hard—if you vow to "go to the gym for two hours" or "run a 10K race," you'll feel achy and uncomfortable and will want to quit. Instead, take it easy. Go for a stroll...try some stretches...splash around in a pool.

Important: During this phase, do not look for results. Do not weigh yourself, take measurements of body parts or worry about whether an exercise is intense enough. Your purpose now is simply to let go of doubts.

WEEKS FOUR THROUGH SIX...

•**Experiment.** Now take a few weeks to try out all the intriguing activities on the list you made previously. Hike in the woods, go ice-skating, rent an aerobics video, try the Pilates class at a friend's club.

Helpful: Many gyms and recreation centers let guests pay by the visit or buy a one-week pass rather than committing right away to (and paying for) a year-long membership. *As you experiment...*

•**Identify favorite activities.** Keep track of what's fun and what's not, looking for patterns. Do you prefer working out at home, or are you inspired by the discipline of going to a health club? Do you like exercising alone or with others? Indoors or outdoors? Consider ways to enhance your enjoyment—for instance, by listening to a portable music player as you walk, watching a movie while using the Stairmaster or buying a new exercise outfit. Within a few weeks, you'll know what you like and what you don't like.

WEEK SEVEN AND BEYOND...

•**Commit.** Now that you've found some enjoyable activities, it's time to decide on a minimum number of workouts you'll do per week—perhaps two or three—and commit to never going below that minimum. Whenever possible, do more than the minimum. Even when you're traveling, you can fit in a half-hour walk or do some yoga poses in your hotel room.

•**Appreciate your progress.** As your exercise habit becomes more ingrained, notice the many positive changes it brings. You feel more energized and less stressed. You sleep more soundly. Your clothes fit better, your weight is easier to control and your posture is straighter. Your muscles are stronger, and everyday tasks are easier. You feel proud of yourself and more in control of your health. Let these benefits serve as reminders of the many reasons why you now love to exercise.

NEW WAYS TO WORK OUT

To keep your workouts fun and fresh, try some activities that you've never done before. *Options to consider...*

•**Core training.** The muscles in the center of your torso, which keep you balanced and support your spine, can be strengthened using equipment developed for this purpose.

Examples: The bosu is an inflated half-sphere that challenges core muscles as you stand on it...the kettlebell is a weighted iron ball with a handle to grip while doing various twists, lunges and other moves. Such equipment usually is available at gyms.

Best: Ask a trainer to help you develop a program using the apparatus.

•**Spinning.** Exercise on a stationary bike, led by an instructor, usually is done to music that fits the pace of the cycling.

•**Video games.** You can do these at home using a game console and your television. In Dance Dance Revolution, you stand on a special mat and move your feet in time to music, following visual cues to perform a series of specific steps. In Wii Fit, you stand on a balance board and get feedback on your technique as you do yoga, strength training, aerobics and balance games.

•**Zumba.** This fusion of Latin rhythms and easy-to-follow dance moves creates a fun fitness workout. For classes near you, visit *www.zumba.com.*

Cold Water for Workouts

Is it best to drink cold water during workouts?

Yes. According to new research, drinking cold water during exercise helps regulate internal body temperature. In the study, 45 physically active men, average age 30, did 60-minute strength and cardiovascular workouts. When they drank water chilled to 39°F in a refrigerator, their core body temperature increased only 2.2% as a result of the exercise, compared with a 3.1% increase when they drank water at room temperature. Elevated core temperature can contribute to fatigue and dehydration.

Amanda Carlson-Phillips, RD, vice president, nutrition and research, Exos, Phoenix.

Stay-in-Bed Workout That Gets Results

Genie Tartell, DC, RN, a sports chiropractor based in Kingston, New York, who was team chiropractor for the New York Reebok aerobic team. She has been a guest on *The View*, CNBC, Fox News, WOR radio and various national radio shows.

People who can't sleep come up with all sorts of crazy ideas—and some great ones, too. For instance, how about a workout that you can do right in your bed? This is not a gentle routine that involves wiggling one toe and then another and taking deep breaths in between... or even an interlude of vigorous romance...but rather a real exercise program that gets your blood circulating, builds muscle and strengthens your core—all without getting out of your bed!

The "Get Fit in Bed" workout is the brainchild of Ted Kavanau, the founding senior producer of CNN. Having a difficult time falling asleep, he did what comes naturally to insomniacs—he tried to find an activity that would make him tired enough to sleep. He began exercising...in bed. An avid fitness enthusiast with a background in martial arts and boxing, Kavanau adapted some of the exercises he did at the gym for the soft surface of a mattress and then added a few yoga and Pilates moves. Before long, he noticed that he had more endurance, his muscle mass was increasing, his mood was good—and, yes, he was sleeping like a baby.

ADJUSTED BY A CHIROPRACTOR

Kavanau took his routine to Genie Tartell, DC, RN, a registered nurse and practicing chiropractor, and asked her to fine-tune the routine for safety. Working with patients of different ages and a variety of health issues, Dr. Tartell tweaked the exercise plan, eliminating moves that might cause any injuries and refining many of the others to accomplish practical efficiency.

According to Dr. Tartell, the new workout plan was a hit. "My arthritic patients found that they were getting out of bed in the morning without feeling stiff, while others who hated exercise were now exercising in bed while watching the news," she said.

Kavanau and Dr. Tartell collaborated on a book, appropriately entitled *Get Fit In Bed*, which provides instruction on 42 different exercises for a variety of abilities. Here Dr. Tartell shares the beginner level program. The routine is organized into exercises to do on your back...on your stomach...on your left side...and on your right side. There are modifications for people with particular physical challenges. The exercises can be done at your own pace and, as you get stronger and fitter, you can increase the number of reps and the speed at which they're performed.

THE STARTER PROGRAM

Always begin your "Get Fit in Bed" routine with a basic gentle stretch. Lie on your back, arms down by your sides. Open and close your hands several times. Then extend your arms above your head, stretching like a cat...and lengthen your legs, one at a time, extending each from the hip. Fan your toes, one foot at a time, and then point your feet (together) toward your head and then away from it several times. This stretching should feel good, like you're waking up your muscles.

Minimal crunch: Lie on your back, arms at your sides, and then tighten your stomach muscles while inhaling. Slowly raise your head and shoulders very slightly (maybe an inch) off the bed, exhaling as you do so. Hold this position for a second or two and then slowly drop your head and shoulders to the bed. Repeat five times.

The bridge: Lie on your back with your knees bent and feet flat on the bed, arms at your sides. Tighten the muscles in your buttocks while slowly lifting your pelvis toward the ceiling. Aim to bring your pelvis and thighs into a straight line, at about a 45-degree angle to your knees. Hold this position for a slow count of 10 (about 20 seconds) and then gently drop back to the bed. Repeat five times.

Crunch: Lie on your back with your knees bent and feet flat on the bed, arms at your sides. Using your abdominal muscles, bring your knees up toward your chest and extend your arms so that your hands reach toward your knees, continuing to bring your upper body closer to your knees. *Note:* Do not pull up with your neck! Lower your upper body halfway down toward the bed. Hold for a slow count of 10 (about 20 seconds). Now repeat five times before lowering your upper body all the way back down to the prone position.

Elbow-knee piston: Lie on your back. Put your hands underneath your head, fingers laced, and bend your knees so that your feet rest flat on the mattress. Raise your bent legs in alternating motions, bringing your left elbow and right knee toward each other—then, as you bring them back down, bring your right elbow and left knee toward each other, raising your upper body to bring knee and elbow as close together as you can. As you get more proficient, increase your speed so that it becomes a pumping motion. Repeat each left/right combination three to six times.

Bicycle with crunches: Similar to the previous exercise, for this one you again lie on your back, arms at your sides. Start with your legs flat on the bed, then raise them and begin moving them as if you were pedaling a bicycle. At the same time, raise your body in a crunch-like position (using your abdominal muscles) and begin "throwing punches" at your feet in sync with your leg movements. Repeat the cycle of left/right punches with corresponding

pedaling five times—your goal is to do a total of 10 punches, five with each hand.

For these next two exercises, turn over onto your stomach...

Forearm-supported body lift: Lie on your stomach, palms flat and under your shoulders, elbows bent in an acute angle. Push off your hands and lift your upper body off the bed, eyes facing forward. Hold this position for two seconds then return to the original position. Repeat five more times.

Cobra: Lie on your stomach, elbows bent, and hands placed flat on the bed in line with your shoulders. Straighten your arms to lift your upper body while curving it back like a cobra—if you're unable to straighten your arms fully, just push up as far as you can. (A soft mattress may limit your ability to get full extension of the arms.) Hold this "up" position for a slow count of 10 and then slowly return to starting position. Repeat just twice for a total of three. *Tip:* Try this exercise with deeper breathing to improve relaxation.

The beauty of this exercise program is that it can be adapted in a variety of ways to fit into your life and can be done as an early morning and/or evening workout. It provides an easy way to work out while traveling, for instance, or (as in Kavanau's case) a good way to put your awake time in the middle of the night to good use.

Work Out for Well-Being, Not Weight Loss

Women who exercised to lose weight spent significantly less time working out than those who exercised to improve their sense of well-being and/or reduce stress.

Effective: For motivation, think of exercise as a way to feel good...and select physical activities that you enjoy.

Michelle Segar, PhD, MPH, director, Sport, Health and Activity Research and Policy Center at the University of Michigan, Ann Arbor and leader of a study of 156 women.

10 Easy Ways to Sneak Exercise Into Your Day

Carol Krucoff is a registered yoga therapist at Duke Integrative Medicine in Durham, North Carolina, where she creates individualized yoga programs for people with health challenges. She is coauthor with her husband, Mitchell Krucoff, MD, of *Healing Moves: How to Cure, Relieve, and Prevent Common Ailments with Exercise.*

Getting the recommended 30 minutes of exercise a day can be challenging during the cold, dark days of winter. But the good news is that you don't have to work out for a half-hour straight to boost your health. New guidelines from the American Heart Association and the American College of Sports Medicine state that three 10-minute bouts of moderate-intensity physical activity (such as a brisk walk) can be just as effective as exercising for 30 minutes straight. And other evidence suggests that even shorter periods of activity—in fact, every step you take—adds up to better health.

Don't let wintry weather freeze your exercise plans. *Try these simple strategies to slip exercise into your day...*

1. Break the elevator/escalator habit. Climbing stairs is a great way to strengthen your heart, muscles and bones. The Harvard Alumni Health Study, which followed 11,130 men (mean age 58 at the beginning of the study) for about 20 years, found that those who climbed 20 to 34 floors per week had about a 30% lower risk of stroke. Take the stairs at every opportunity and even look for ways to add extra flights, such as using the bathroom on a different floor. If you must take an elevator up a tall building, get off a few flights early and walk.

2. Use muscle, not machines. In our push-button world, we expend about 300 to 700 fewer calories per day than did our grandparents, who had to do things like chop wood and fetch water. Drop the "labor saving" mentality, and embrace opportunities to activate your life. Use a rake instead of a leaf blower... wash your car by hand...get up and change the TV channel.

3. Walk to a coworker's office instead of sending an e-mail. William Haskell, PhD, calculated, in *The Journal of the American Medical Association,* that the energy expenditure lost by writing e-mails for two minutes every hour for eight hours per day five days a week—instead of two minutes of slow walking around the office to deliver messages—adds up to the equivalent of 1.1 pounds of fat in one year and 11 pounds of fat in 10 years.

4. Take exercise breaks. Energize your body with movement instead of caffeine by turning your coffee break into a "walk break." Every hour or two, get up and walk around or stretch.

5. Wait actively. If you're forced to wait for an airplane, hairdresser, dentist, doctor, restaurant table, etc., take a walk. To boost the calorie burn of your walk, move purposefully—as if you're late for a meeting—rather than just strolling along.

6. Do the housework boogie. Play lively music when you're doing household chores, and dance off extra calories by moving to the beat.

7. Try aerobic shopping. Take a lap or two around the mall or grocery store before you go into a store or put anything in your cart.

8. Socialize actively. Instead of sitting and talking (or eating) with friends and/or family, do something active, such as bowling, playing Ping-Pong, shooting baskets or dancing.

9. Install a chin-up bar in a convenient doorway. Whenever you walk through, do a pull-up or simply "hang out" and stretch. Chin-up bars are available at sporting-goods stores and online for less than $20.

10. Practice "phone fitness." Stretch, walk or climb stairs while you're talking on your cell phone or cordless phone.

Exercise—When Less Is More

Maureen MacDonald, PhD, professor, department of kinesiology, McMaster University, Hamilton, Ontario, Canada.

How many times have you said, "I don't have time to exercise"? After you read this story, that excuse won't work anymore.

A new study found that just three 30-minute sessions a week of a fancy-sounding type of activity called Modified High-Intensity Interval Training (MHIT) is an effective way to strengthen your cardiovascular system, which can lead to increased fitness, strength and weight loss. (It's a lot like regular interval training, which you've surely heard of, but the intervals are even shorter.)

If it sounds hard, don't sweat it. Researchers found that even cardiac rehab patients can handle MHIT—and gain from it.

GOING "ALL OUT"

The gist of MHIT is that it requires just three 30-minute sessions a week, ideally spaced a few days apart. So each workout is quick, but you work very hard during those short spans. Beyond a five-minute warm-up and a five-minute cool-down, it always involves some sort of aerobic activity, generally running, cycling or rowing. You alternate going at an easy pace for one minute with going "all-out" the following minute, repeating that two-minute pattern 10 times in a row.

Researchers in Canada were curious to see if a three-month regimen of short bursts of MHIT might help people who were in cardiac rehab (for either heart disease or heart attack) strengthen their cardiovascular systems more than they would by following a longer, standard exercise program done at a more moderate pace.

Here's how the study worked: Researchers placed 22 male cardiac patients in either an MHIT program or a standard "moderate endurance" program. Both groups focused on stationary cycling, but the MHIT group did three weekly 20-minute sessions that consisted of the intervals described above, while the traditional exercise group did three longer weekly sessions (30 to 50 minutes) at a consistent moderate pace the entire time. Each group did a five-minute warm-up and a five-minute cool-down before and after each exercise session.

The findings: By the end of three months, both groups of exercisers showed virtually equal improvement. Blood flow improved by 41% in the MHIT group and 42% in the endurance group, and oxygen consumption improved 27% in the MHIT group and 19% in the endurance group. But the interesting part is that the MHIT group did it with just 90 total minutes of exercise per week, while it took the moderate exercise group a total of 120 to 180 minutes a week to achieve the same goal.

To discuss the study results, I called the study author, Maureen MacDonald, PhD, professor in the kinesiology department at McMaster University in Hamilton, Ontario. She explained that when your heart is forced to work at a higher-intensity level during MHIT, you can reap the same benefits in less time. I was surprised that cardiac rehab patients could handle such intensity, but Dr. MacDonald said that MHIT actually does not put any more stress on the heart than the standard exercise routine, because the "rest" intervals allow the heart to recover, so the heart doesn't get overworked.

ADDING MHIT TO YOUR REGIMEN

If you're interested in trying MHIT yourself but you have a serious health condition, Dr. MacDonald advises that you check with your doctor first. (Dr. MacDonald did not include people with chronic heart failure in her study due to the severity of the condition.) Otherwise, why not give MHIT a shot? MHIT needs to be done only three days a week, so you still can do strength training and stretching on other days of the week.

To try MHIT, choose your favorite aerobic exercise—whether it's jogging, cycling or rowing—and follow these guidelines from Dr. MacDonald...

• **Warm up for five minutes by lightly doing whatever aerobic activity you choose, so your breathing is light.**

• **For the one-minute intensity cycles, either increase your speed, increase your incline (such as running uphill) or increase the resistance if you are using gym equipment such as a stationary bicycle or elliptical machine.** If you can keep track of your heart rate, either through a monitor that you wear or through a monitor on the machine that you're using, increase your heart rate to 80% to 90% of your maximum rate. To determine your maximum heart rate, subtract your age from 220. It should be very difficult to carry on a conversation at this pace, and your muscles should feel like they are working very hard.

• **For the one-minute recovery cycles, do not stop the activity, but simply slow your speed or reduce your incline or resistance back to normal.** Your heart rate should be about 10% of your maximum (or about your "warm-up" pace). You should be able to carry on a conversation easily at this pace.

After 10 of these two-minute cycles, cool down for about five minutes (or until your heart rate goes below 100 beats per minute) by lightly continuing the aerobic exercise to bring your heart rate down.

Just Two Minutes of Exercise Boosts Mood

Just two minutes of activity raises your heart rate and increases the body's production of neurotransmitters such as norepinephrine, dopamine and serotonin—the same substances increased by antidepressants.

John J. Ratey, MD, associate professor of psychiatry, Harvard Medical School, Boston, and author of *Spark: The Revolutionary New Science of Exercise and the Brain*, quoted in *Prevention*.

Can You Exercise When You're Sick?

It's okay to exercise when you have a runny nose or sore throat. Don't exercise if you have a fever, shortness of breath, chest congestion, body aches, diarrhea or vomiting—or you feel dizzy or light-headed when you stand up.

Keith Veselik, MD, medical director of primary care, Loyola University Health System, Maywood, Illinois.

To Lose Weight...Eat More—And Other Proven Ways to Drop Pounds

Jonathan Bailor, a health-and-fitness researcher based in the Seattle area who analyzed more than 10,000 pages of academic research related to diet, exercise and weight loss for his book *The Smarter Science of Slim: Scientific Proof.*

There is a science to weight loss, but the facts often are obscured by the myths. For example, the calories-in, calories-out theory says that for every 3,500 calories you lose, you drop a pound of fat. If you follow this logic, a 150-pound woman who reduced her daily caloric intake by 100 calories (the amount in less than one cup of reduced-fat milk) for 10 years would give up 365,000 calories—and would weigh only 46 pounds!

Despite what you've heard, calories are not all that matter...they're not all the same...and the government's dietary guidelines are not effective for weight control.

WHAT REALLY WORKS...

Eat more to lose weight. It's true. People who consume more food gain less weight than those who cut calories—but only as long as the calories come from the right foods.

Example: When researchers at the University of Pennsylvania compared the effects of higher- and lower-calorie diets, they found that people who ate more lost 200% more weight.

A diet high in high-quality foods (such as protein-rich seafood, nuts and seeds and non-starchy vegetables, such as celery, asparagus and salad greens) increases satiety, the ability of calories to fill you up and keep you full. The same foods are less likely to be stored as body fat than, say, processed foods, and they're more likely to be burned off with your normal metabolism.

People who eat less to lose weight usually fail because the body interprets calorie restriction as starvation. For self-protection, it hangs on to body fat and instead utilizes muscle tissue for energy. Up to 70% of the weight that people lose on a low-cal diet actually is muscle tissue, not fat.

When we eat more—but smarter—we are satisfied…eat only the number of calories that we really need…and provide our body with an abundance of nutrition. This enables us to sustainably burn body fat.

• **Focus on protein.** Protein is a high-satiety nutrient that triggers the release of hormones that send I've had enough signals to the brain. In a University of Washington study, participants were allowed an unlimited amount of calories as long as 30% of those calories came from protein.

Result: They consumed 441 fewer calories a day—without feeling hungry.

Protein is less likely to be converted to fat. When you eat an egg omelet or a chicken breast, about one-third of the protein calories are burned during digestion…another one-third are burned when the liver converts protein to glucose (a process called gluconeogenesis).

Compare this to what happens when you eat bread or other starchy foods. About 70% of those calories can be stored as fat.

Recommended: Get one-third of your calories from protein—in the form of seafood, poultry, meat or nonfat dairy, such as plain Greek yogurt or cottage cheese.

• **Don't neglect fiber.** This isn't new advice, but most people still don't get enough fiber—or understand why it helps.

The fiber in plant foods isn't digested or absorbed. Instead, it takes up space in the digestive tract…and makes you fill up faster and stay full longer. This is why you will feel more satisfied when you eat, say, 200 calories worth of celery instead of 200 calories worth of candy. The celery takes up about 30 times more space.

You don't have to "count" fiber grams. As long as you get about one-third of total calories from nonstarchy vegetables (discussed previously), you'll get enough.

• **Don't believe the claims about grains.** Whole-wheat bread, oatmeal, brown rice and other grains will not help you lose weight.

Reason: The calories in grains are aggressive, which means that they're more likely to be stored as fat than the calories that you get from protein or nonstarchy carbohydrates. Grains—even whole grains—are rapidly converted to glucose (blood sugar) in the body. The rapid rise in glucose is followed by an equally rapid drop-off. This stimulates the appetite and causes you to crave more calories.

Also, fast-rising glucose is hard for the body to handle. It responds by attempting to rid itself of glucose—by storing it in fat cells.

• **Eat fat.** It's true that fat has about twice as many calories as protein or carbohydrates, but that would matter only if the calories-in, calories-out equation had anything to do with weight loss—which it doesn't.

Decades ago, doctors encouraged Americans to consume fewer calories from fat.

Result: The average person got heavier, not leaner. Experts now agree that people who consume more fat are no more likely to be overweight or obese than those who eat less—if anything, the people who eat less fat are more likely to gain weight.

Recommended: Get about one-third of your calories from fats, including olive and canola oils (monunsaturated fats that lower your risk for heart disease) and the fats in meats, poultry and fish.

• **Drink a lot of green tea.** You will naturally burn more fat when you drink more water. If you get much of this water in the form of green tea, you will do even better. The polyphenols in green tea are among the healthiest antioxidants ever discovered. These compounds, along with the caffeine in tea (about one-fifth the amount in coffee), increase fat metabolism. If you drink decaffeinated tea, you still will burn more fat than you would just by drinking water.

Recommended: Between five and 15 cups of green tea daily. For maximum efficiency, put all the tea bags you need for the day in hot water. Let the tea brew for a few minutes, and then drink the tea throughout the day like iced tea...or put it in the microwave if you prefer hot tea.

Lose Fat While You Shower?

Denis Richard, PhD, is director of research at the Quebec Heart and Lung Institute Research Centre and Laval University Interdisciplinary Group in Obesity Research in Quebec, Canada. He also is the lead author of a recent study on brown fat published in the journal *Frontiers in Bioscience*.

Can taking a cold shower help the body burn more fat? Is a cold rinse a good way to help control weight?

Despite what you may have read on the Web or in other media, the short answer is no. Or at least it would have to be a very long and very cold shower—and even then, the effects on weight or body composition would be negligible.

Here's why: Our bodies have two different types of fat. So-called white fat stores energy and is present in excess in people who are overweight. Brown fat, which is abundant in newborns but diminishes with age, produces energy and helps maintain body temperature. When activated, brown fat burns white fat as fuel—and cold exposure does indeed stimulate an increase in the amount and activity of brown fat. However, for that stimulation to occur, you would have to be exposed to cold nearly to the point of shivering for some uncomfortable minutes—and once the cold exposure stopped, the thermogenic (heat- and

energy-producing) effects of the brown fat activity also would cease. So, you would get very little benefit in terms of fat-burning from that unpleasantly chilly shower.

Someday, research on brown fat may lead to new options in the prevention and treatment of obesity. But for now, the bottom line is that you can take a cold rinse at the end of your shower if you find it invigorating—but don't count on that to help you burn fat.

Want to Get Slim Fast? How Not to Fail at Weight Loss

Bill Phillips, author of the best seller *Transformation: The Mindset You Need, The Body You Want, The Life You Deserve.* He is based in Golden, Colorado.

How many people do you know who have tried...and tried...and tried to lose weight but just can't do it?

It just might be that you are one of them—and if so, you have plenty of company. In a recent year more than 50 million Americans went on diets—and the vast majority (95%) of those men and women are in no better shape today. As anyone who has tried losing weight knows, it requires lots of planning and attitude adjustment if you want to succeed. Happily we had an opportunity to speak recently with Bill Phillips, author of the perennial best seller *Body for LIFE* and the book *Transformation: The Mindset You Need, The Body You Want, The Life You Deserve.* We asked him to share his proven techniques for getting past the traps that catch people when they're trying to shed pounds and gain better health.

THREE SECRETS OF SUCCESS

Phillips said that if you want to lose weight, the first thing you need to do is reframe the idea. Instead of thinking about dieting, realize that you are about to transform your life for the better. Since losing weight benefits your entire life on many levels—not just when you get on the scale—he encourages people to come up with a holistic plan that encompasses changes for your mind, body and soul. And this is not as hard as it sounds!

Phillips said he has found three factors critical to success...

- **Maintain a positive perspective.**
- **Stay motivated.**
- **Stay focused.**

These concepts can seem so basic, and yet so big at the same time, that it is easy to stop before you start. *But Phillips knows how you can avoid that...*

The Trap: Fad diets and other restrictive plans. Whether it's eating mostly protein or only cabbage soup, fad and crash diets are nutritionally unsound and totally lacking in enjoyment, making them ultimately doomed to failure—few people can live long-term with so many restrictions.

Instead: Plan for a new way of life. "Transformation is a process of changing the whole person to become healthier, happier, lighter, more energized and aware," Phillips said, suggesting you figure out what dietary changes you need to make for your new life rather than putting yourself on a "diet." Instead of trying to eat foods that you don't like, learn how to make healthy versions of the meals that you do like. He explains, "My favorite dinner foods are chicken enchiladas, spaghetti and meatballs and homemade thin crust pizza. The key is I've learned how to make these meals so they're high in nutrients, low in calories and as delicious as ever." (These and other recipes can be found for free at *www.bodybuilding.com/fun/healthy-recipe-database.html.*)

The Trap: Lacking focus and a goal. Without a specific focus—a clearly defined goal—most everyone will have trouble staying on the straight and narrow path. Phillips said, "The mind seems to work somewhat like a GPS system in the modern car. If you don't program in the specific coordinates of where you want to go, it can't help you get there."

Instead: Be clear about where you're starting and where you're going. As soon as you identify a target that can be objectively measured—such as becoming 30 pounds lighter in 18 weeks—it's like you turn the headlights on

after driving all night in the dark. Think about that GPS system again and how it's akin to the human mind—when we are crystal clear about where we are going, it's remarkable how it will help us get there.

The Trap: Excuses, excuses. If you're carrying around a mental list of reasons why your plan won't work—such as I don't have time to exercise or cook healthy foods or I'm too old for this—you can be sure that you'll fail.

Instead: Focus on the true reward. Phillips encourages people trying to lose weight to look inward for the reasons why. "One deeply purposeful reason will override 100 excuses," states Phillips. Superficial reasons, such as, I don't want to be embarrassed at the reunion next month, or wanting to look better than someone else, may not have the power to inspire over the long term. Phillips finds that when people connect with the deeper reasons for transforming their health, it can be like flipping a switch...where they go from struggling to maintaining new, positive habits to an almost instant and somewhat effortless compliance. Many people who have a health crisis experience this jolt instantly—they realize that if they don't nurture their well-being and cut out the unhealthy patterns of action, they're not going to be there for their kids, grandkids, friends or coworkers. "The more 'other-centered' people's reasons for making the decision to change, the more power in the near and long-term they have," Phillips finds.

Tip: Write your reasons for wanting to lose weight on an index card, and keep it with you. The next time you are tempted to dip a chip at a party or skip your morning workout, take a look at your note to remind yourself why it's better to just say no.

The Trap: Constantly weighing yourself. Amazingly, your body weight can fluctuate up to several pounds over the course of one day—and most of that is water weight. Not losing as you expect or, worse, gaining weight one day can throw you off ...some people think, why bother? and immediately sabotage their success.

Instead: Step off the scale. Weigh yourself only once a week—preferably on the same day at the same time each week. In the interim, pay attention to how you feel (lighter? more energetic?) and how your clothes fit.

The Trap: Everyone else is indulging! Without a strong and supportive group of people around you, it's way too easy to get off track—bad habits are contagious!

Instead: Enlist help from friends and family. Tell people you love what you are trying to do and ask for support, encouragement and help. Invite an upbeat friend or neighbor to join you in regular walks or bike rides—it'll be more fun and will motivate you to stick with the program. Join a community weight-loss support group or take part in free support forums at *www.bodybuilding.com.* "You don't have to completely disconnect from friends who haven't yet made the decision to be healthy, but it's important to have contact with at least one other person each day who's making the kind of positive, challenging changes that you are making."

The Trap: Getting discouraged. If you measure your progress by what hasn't happened (you're not thin yet!) rather than what has (your eating habits are getting healthier, your jeans are loose), you are at risk for falling into what Phillips calls "The Void." In this frame of mind, you may convince yourself that you have failed and abandon your transformation journey altogether.

Instead: Invent a game you can win. Forget about pursuing perfection, and focus on making progress. List very specific steps you can take today or this week that move you in the direction of your meaningful and specific goals.

Example: "Today I will eat six nutrient-rich, calorie-sparse meals and work out for 30 minutes."

The big secret to weight-loss success is sustainability, says Phillips. Take joy in your small improvements each day and week—such as your new ways of eating and exercising and the energy, self-confidence and sense of well-being that comes with them. There's only one real way to fail, he adds—and that's to stop trying.

"Small" Secret to Outwitting a Big Appetite

Devina Wadhera, PhD, research professor, department of psychology at Arizona State University in Tempe and lead author of a study on food piece size and satiety presented at a recent annual meeting of the Society for the Study of Ingestive Behavior in Zurich.

A recent study outlines a simple cut-food-up-and-eat-less strategy that may work as a painless weight-loss technique for dieters. The 301 study volunteers fasted overnight and skipped breakfast before the experiment began. Then they each were given a bagel and cream cheese. One group of participants got bagels that were whole...the other group got identical bagels, except that theirs had been cut into four pieces. After eating as much of their bagels as they wanted, they spent 20 minutes filling out questionnaires about food preferences—a delaying tactic, because it takes about 20 minutes after eating for the brain to get the message that the stomach is full. Next, each participant was invited to eat as much as desired of a complimentary lunch that included a turkey sandwich, veggies with dressing, crackers with meat and cheese, mozzarella sticks, pasta, potato salad and a cupcake.

Fascinating findings: Compared with participants who had received whole bagels, those whose bagels had been cut up ate 8% less of their bagels—but the real revelation was that they also ate 40% less of the big lunch! Apparently, the cut-up bagels had done a much better job of satisfying participants' appetites, so when offered additional food later, they were less tempted by it.

Especially in this era of out-of-control portion sizes, it's smart for us to make regular use of this simple tactic—cut up food to make it seem more plentiful and thus more satisfying. We have nothing to lose but weight.

Forbidden Foods That Promote Weight Loss

Don't ban foods you like when dieting. Putting specific foods off limits creates a constant craving for them and makes a diet more likely to fail.

Also: Many foods that dieters try to avoid may help with weight loss.

Examples: Some breads contain complex carbohydrates, which increase brain chemicals that reduce overeating…pasta's high fluid content keeps you feeling fuller longer…potatoes contain a fiber that burns fat…dark chocolate satisfies a common craving, so eating moderate amounts can make a binge less likely.

Bottom line: Portion control and a focus on nutrient-rich foods lead to successful weight loss.

D. Milton Stokes, PhD,MPH, certified registered dietitian-nutritionist, director, global health and nutrition outreach, Monsanto Company, quoted in *Prevention*.

Foods That Rev Up Your Metabolism— Drop Those Extra Pounds for Good!

Ridha Arem, MD, an endocrinologist, director of the Texas Thyroid Institute in Houston. He is a former chief of endocrinology at Houston's Ben Taub General Hospital and is the author of *The Thyroid Solution Diet*. AremWellness.com

Forget about calories! Most people who are trying to lose weight worry too much about calories and not enough about the actual cause of those extra pounds.

The real culprit: Out-of-balance hormones.

Best approach for controlling weight: A diet that rebalances the body's hormones. Carefully chosen foods and food combinations rebalance levels and/or efficiency of metabolism-regulating hormones, such as ghrelin, leptin and thyroid hormone. You'll burn more calories, and your body will be less likely to store calories as fat. *Here's how…*

TWEAKING THE BEST DIETS

Hands down, the Mediterranean diet is one of the healthiest diets out there. With its emphasis on plant-based foods (such as vegetables, fruits, grains and nuts) and healthful fats (from fatty fish and olive oil), it is good for your heart and helps control blood sugar levels.

But for more efficient weight loss, you need to go a step further. That's where the Protein-Rich Oriental Diet, developed by Korean researchers, enters the picture. With its heavy focus on high-protein foods, this diet has been found to provide twice the weight loss offered by calorie restriction alone.

To achieve and maintain an optimal body weight: The diet I designed includes elements of both these diets—as well as some important additional tweaks such as timing your meals (see "Timing Matters" on the next page) and consuming a mix of proteins in order to get the full complement of amino acids, which is essential for increasing metabolism and controlling hunger. On my diet, you will eat a combination of at least two proteins, good fats and vegetables at each meal. *For example…*

● **Fish, turkey and chicken** contain all of the essential amino acids that are in red meat, but with fewer calories and less saturated fat. They're particularly rich in arginine, an amino acid that increases the speed at which your body burns calories.

My advice: Aim for six to eight ounces of these foods as the primary protein for dinner. You also can include these foods at breakfast and lunch as one of your protein choices.

● **Reduced-fat cottage cheese, ricotta, yogurt and goat cheese.** Certain forms of dairy are high in branched-chain amino acids, which suppress appetite and increase the ability of mitochondria (the energy-producing components of cells) to burn fat.

My advice: Each day, eat about a half-cup of low-fat or nonfat dairy as a protein.

• **High-protein beans, lentils and grains, such as black beans, kidney beans, quinoa and brown rice.** Eat one of these protein sources (three-fourths cup to one cup) at lunch—usually combined with a small serving of fish or lean meat. In addition to packing plenty of protein and fiber, these foods provide large amounts of amino acids that will help you get fitter and have more energy.

• **Egg whites** contain all of the amino acids that you need for efficient weight loss, and they are my favorite choice as a protein for breakfast. An egg-white omelet with onions, mushrooms and other vegetables can be prepared in just a few minutes. Limit your intake of egg yolks due to their cholesterol.

LOW-GLYCEMIC CARBS

Carbohydrates that are digested quickly—mainly refined and processed foods such as juices, white rice and French fries—increase insulin and fat storage. Carbohydrates with a lower glycemic score are absorbed more slowly and don't cause unhealthy changes in insulin or fat storage.

Good choices: Whole oats, chickpeas and fruit (see below) at breakfast and lunch, and vegetables at each meal.

MORE FIBER

The fiber in such foods as beans and vegetables reduces appetite and slows digestion, important for preventing insulin "spikes." Research shows that people of normal weight tend to eat significantly more fiber than those who are overweight or obese.

For efficient weight loss: Get 35 g of fiber daily.

Fruit is also a good source of fiber. Just be sure that you choose fresh fruit that's low in natural sugar (fructose).

Good choices: Raspberries, strawberries, papayas, apples and cranberries. Avoid fruit at dinner to make it the lowest glycemic meal.

GREEN TEA

Green tea is high in epigallocatechin gallate (EGCG), a substance that can decrease the accumulation of body fat. It also increases insulin sensitivity and improves an obesity-related condition known as metabolic syndrome. Drink a few cups every day. Do not sweeten the tea with honey or other sweeteners—they are among the main causes of high insulin and weight gain.

FISH OIL SUPPLEMENTS

The omega-3 fatty acids in fish increase the rate at which calories are burned. However, even if you eat fish every day, it doesn't contain enough omega-3s for long-term weight control.

Solution: Take a daily supplement with 600 mg of EPA and 400 mg of DHA—the main types of omega-3s. Check first with your doctor if you take blood thinners or diabetes medication, since fish oil may interact with these drugs.

NOT JUST FOR WEIGHT LOSS

A hormone-balancing eating plan can rev up your metabolism even if you don't need to lose weight, giving you more energy and mental focus. If you aren't overweight and you follow this eating plan, you may lose a pound or two, but mostly you'll just feel better.

TIMING MATTERS!

When you eat is almost as important as what you eat…

• **Plan on eating four or five daily meals**—breakfast between 6 am and 8 am…an optional (and light) late-morning snack…lunch between 11 am and 12:30 pm…a mid-afternoon snack…and supper between 5 pm and 7 pm.

• **Plan your meals so that you get more protein at supper.** It will stimulate the release of growth hormone, which burns fat while you sleep.

• **Avoid all food three hours before bedtime.** Eating late in the evening causes increases in blood sugar and insulin that can lead to weight gain—even if you consume a lower-calorie diet (1,200 to 1,500 calories a day).

10

Look Great, Feel Great

Do-It-Yourself Face-Lift

If you've got facial wrinkles that you would like to reduce but you don't want to get Botox injections or a surgical face-lift, there's a do-it-yourself option that's far less invasive and far less expensive.

With a technique known as facial acupressure (similar to acupuncture but performed without needles), you can take up to five to 10 years off your appearance—and perhaps even improve your overall health in the process.

Sound far-fetched?

I've treated hundreds of patients who were contemplating face-lifts but found success with acupressure.

Bonus: Unlike Botox or surgery, acupressure won't give you a tight, frozen or pulled-back appearance. The results are softer and more natural.

WHY ACUPRESSURE?

Acupressure is based on a Chinese healing technique that involves pressing or kneading key points on the body to stimulate energy flow, known as Qi (pronounced chee), through invisible pathways called meridians. It can be used to relax or tone muscles, boost circulation and even improve digestion.

The conventional view: From the Western medical perspective, wrinkles are formed by changes in the skin's composition, thickness and elasticity as well as continuous muscle activity—for example, forehead wrinkles may appear after years of furrowing your eyebrows or squinting. As a result, the skin covering the muscle creases, eventually creating a wrinkle.

Chinese medicine has a different perspective. For example, specific meridians (that correspond to organ systems, such as those for the "Liver" and "Gallbladder") are believed to

Shellie Goldstein, LAc, a licensed acupuncturist, esthetician and certified Chinese herbologist who maintains a private practice in New York City and Wainscott, New York (*HamptonsAcupuncture.com*). One of the first acupuncturists to work in hospitals and health-care facilities in New York state, Goldstein is the author of *Your Best Face Now: Look Younger in 20 Days with the Do-It-Yourself Acupressure Facelift*.

affect certain body parts, but they don't always seem to correlate. For instance, a meridian located at the junction between your thumb and index finger corresponds to the head—rubbing that area can reduce headaches and, yes, wrinkles.

DO-IT-YOURSELF ROUTINES

To help reduce wrinkles and puffiness, use the following routines each day until you are satisfied with the results and then as needed…

● **Forehead wrinkles.**

What to do: Begin at the top of your right foot, in the junction between your big and second toes. (This point is called "Liver 3.") Using medium to firm (but not painful) pressure, massage the point in a clockwise circle 10 times. (If you have arthritic fingers, use your knuckle instead.) Repeat on left foot.

Next, move to the back side of your right hand between your right thumb and index finger ("Large Intestine 4"). In a clockwise circular motion, massage this point for 10 rotations. Repeat on the left hand.

Then, move to the back of your neck. Place both thumbs where your spine meets the base of your skull and move them two inches to either side until they each land in an indentation ("Gallbladder 20"). Massage clockwise with firm pressure for 10 rotations.

Lastly, move to your face. Place the pad of each index finger a half inch above the center of each eyebrow ("Gallbladder 14"). Massage with medium pressure in 10 clockwise (right to left) circles.

Repeat the entire sequence three times in a single session each day. For deeper wrinkles, do the sequence several times throughout the day. You should notice a reduction in forehead wrinkles within 20 days.

● **Under-eye puffiness** (due to age or allergies). *What to do:* Place your index finger two inches above the inside of your right ankle between the bone and muscle ("Spleen 6"). Do 10 clockwise rotations using medium to firm pressure. Repeat on left leg.

Next, move to the back of your right hand ("Large Intestine 4"), as described earlier, and perform 10 clockwise rotations. Repeat on the left hand.

Then, with your arm at your side, bend your left elbow to make a 90° angle. Pinpoint the area located at the outside edge of the elbow crease, between the bend and the bone ("Large Intestine 11"). Use your index finger to massage 10 times in a clockwise rotation using medium to firm pressure. Repeat on your right elbow.

Lastly, move to your face. Place your right index finger just to the side of your right nostril. Move the finger laterally to a spot directly underneath the center of your eye, in your sinus area ("Stomach 3"). Press in and slightly upward, performing 10 clockwise rotations. Repeat on the left side.

Do the entire sequence three times daily. You should notice a reduction in puffiness under your eyes after a few days.

The Silicon Secret To Better Health And Greater Beauty

Mark A. Stengler, NMD, a naturopathic medical doctor and author of the *Health Revelations* newsletter, author of *The Natural Physician's Healing Therapies,* founder and medical director of the Stengler Center for Integrative Medicine in Encinitas, California, and adjunct associate clinical professor at the National College of Natural Medicine in Portland, Oregon. *MarkStengler.com*

Editor's note: You may not be familiar with silicon (no, it has nothing to do with silicone breast implants), but this mineral is definitely worth getting to know. Why? Silicon can reduce wrinkles and enhance skin luster…add volume to thinning hair…make nails more break-resistant…and build stronger bones and healthier joints, too.

The following special report on silicon comes from Mark A. Stengler, NMD, founder and medical director of the Stengler Center for Integrative Medicine in Encinitas, California, and author of *The Natural Physician's Healing Therapies. Dr. Stengler writes…*

Patients often are surprised when I recommend silicon for their thinning hair or brittle nails. I believe that this mineral is a well-kept

103

secret in the medical world. Note that silicon, the mineral, is different from silicone, the synthetic compound that (in gel form) is used in some medical applications and products, including breast implants.

Silicon is amazing—it's the second most common mineral in the Earth's crust and is found in sand on beaches. While it was once believed to be an inert contaminant, researchers discovered more than a century ago that silicon was concentrated in many of the body's tissues. What's more, silicon plays a role in keeping us healthy by strengthening bone and joint cartilage and maintaining the health of hair, skin and fingernails. *How silicon can help you...*

HEALTH BENEFITS OF SILICON

You may have heard silicon referred to as a "trace mineral," a mineral needed by the body in only very small amounts. But there is growing evidence that silicon could eventually be regarded as a macro mineral, which is required in amounts larger than that provided by food alone.

We have silicon in every cell of our bodies. Concentrations of silicon are highest in bone, connective tissues, skin, fingernails and hair, as well as the trachea, tendons and aorta—tissues that need strength and/or resilience. *Silicon's main role is to enhance the structural integrity of specific tissues, such as...*

• **Collagen.** Scientific evidence points to silicon being involved in the synthesis and "stability" of collagen, the body's chief protein. We need collagen to make most of our organs, bone and the fibrous tissues of the skin, tendons and ligaments. Without adequate collagen production, bones and ligaments weaken and skin tissue is compromised.

• **Joint cartilage.** Collagen and noncollagen proteins are needed to make joint cartilage, the role of which is to protect the joints and enable bones to move freely.

• **Bone.** Silicon is a major constituent of bone-making cells. Concentrations of the mineral are especially high in cells actively forming new bone. The mineral enhances the absorption of calcium, and a lack of silicon reduces the calcium content of bone. High intake of silicon is associated with better bone-mineral density and stronger bones.

Several studies have found that taking supplemental silicon increases the mineral density of bones.

Example: A study of postmenopausal women published in *BMC Musculoskeletal Disorders* found that adding a silicon supplement improved bone-mineral density above and beyond what was achieved with just calcium and vitamin D supplementation.

Skin, hair, fingernails. Several small but promising studies have found that supplemental silicon often can restore a younger- and -healthier-looking appearance. This is probably related to collagen and elastin production. Elastin is a protein that, as the name suggests, gives skin the ability to stretch. One study found that a commercial silicon oral supplement called RegeneMax reduced micro-wrinkle depth by 30%. It also improved the youthful look, or elasticity, of the skin. Other studies have found that silicon supplements can increase the thickness of hair strands and strengthen fingernails, making them more resistant to breaking.

GETTING SILICON INTO YOUR BODY

While silicon was once plentiful in herbs and grains, farming methods have depleted silicon from the ground, so many plant foods are not as rich in silicon as they could be. Because of this, most people have suboptimal levels of silicon. We need 5 grams (g) to 20 g daily of silicon—and the best way to get this amount is to take supplemental silicon.

For those people who have thinning hair or lackluster, aging skin and want a more youthful appearance, I recommend taking 5 mg daily of choline-stabilized orthosilicic acid, which is biologically active and much better absorbed than silicon derived from herbal sources. It is available in liquid and capsule form. If you have severe osteoporosis or osteoarthritis or brittle nails or hair, consider taking 10 mg daily. If your body takes in more silicon than it needs, you excrete the excess (so taking in more than you need at these doses is not a problem).

Brands to try: BioSil by Natural Factors (877-551-2179, *www.NaturalFactors.com* for a store locator)...JarroSil by Jarrow Formulas (310-204-6936, *www.Jarrow.com*)...and Xymogen's RegeneMax (800-647-6100, *www.Xymogen.com*, available through health-care professionals).

There are no side effects, and silicon is safe to take with other medications. Silicon supplements should be avoided by people with chronic kidney disease (excess silicon could result in further kidney damage) and women who are pregnant.

Baggy, Saggy Skin on Your Cheekbones? Send It Packing

Adam J. Scheiner, MD, is a board-certified oculoplastic and facial plastic surgeon in Tampa. He has published numerous scientific papers on eyelid surgery and is an instructor for the American Academy of Ophthalmology. Dr. Scheiner practices at the Tampa Eye & Specialty Surgery Center Clinic and recently discussed festoon removal on *The Dr. Oz Show.*

The word festoons may make you think of festivals or balloons, but they're hardly a reason for celebration. These puffy mounds of saggy, hammocklike skin beneath the lower eyelids can make you look far older or more tired than you might actually be. In some cases, festoons can even interfere with vision—for instance, when you look down to read and find your view blocked by these bags of flesh high on your cheekbones.

Aging contributes to the likelihood of developing festoons...so can a light complexion or genetic predisposition. But the biggest risk factor is sun exposure because ultraviolet rays damage the collagen and elastin fibers that give skin its underlying structure. The many home remedies people try—ice packs, tea bags, chilled cucumber slices placed over the eyes—fail to fix the problem because they cannot repair the damaged fibers. The skin's natural process of regeneration cannot get rid of festoons because normally only the top layer of skin regrows itself. Conventional cosmetic surgery, such as a face-lift or blepharoplasty (eyelid surgery), requires incisions, sometimes

leaves scars and may even make festoons more noticeable.

Breakthrough: A technique called ablative laser skin resurfacing gets rid of festoons by getting rid of the damaged skin and allowing healthy new skin to take its place. Adam J. Scheiner, MD, an oculoplastic surgeon (an ophthalmologist with special training in cosmetic surgery around the eyes) based in Tampa, treats festoons with this 30-minute in-office procedure using a dual-pulsed erbium laser. It's the same type of laser typically used for treating sun damage, wrinkles and precancerous lesions on other areas of the face.

The procedure: Dr. Scheiner explained that local anesthesia is injected to numb the under-eye area...the eyes are numbed with drops and covered with protective lenses. Then pulses of laser are applied to each festoon, removing the skin layer by layer until the deeper layer—where new elastin and collagen fibers grow from the bottom up—is reached. It is the deeper treatment of the laser that allows skin to grow back festoon-free, Dr. Scheiner said.

Recovery: Because the laser seals off blood vessels and nerve endings, postoperative discomfort and bruising are minimal. Dr. Scheiner said that the treated skin initially looks sunburned...after a day or so, it looks like a red, healing blister. For the first day or two, you wear a bandage over the area. For two weeks, you refrain from wearing contact lenses and makeup...and several times a day, you apply a cloth soaked in a mild vinegar solution to prevent infection and follow this with a healing ointment (such as Aquaphor) to lubricate the area. After two weeks, the area looks slightly pinker than usual...pinkness disappears completely within four to five months. Results are permanent, Dr. Scheiner said, provided that you protect your skin against further damage by using sunscreen and sunglasses whenever you are outdoors during daylight.

Festoon removal is considered a cosmetic procedure, so it is not covered by insurance. Fees range from $5,000 to $10,000, depending on the complexity of the case. People who have had radiation to the face or who have used the acne medication *isotretinoin* in the past six months should not have this procedure.

Dr. Scheiner recommended that festoon removal be performed by an oculoplastic surgeon or a physician who has extensive experience with the eyes and ablative laser skin resurfacing. To find a doctor, visit the website of the American Academy of Ophthalmology at *www.aao.org* and in the "Subspeciality" box, click on "Plastics/Reconstructive."

Splotchy Skin? The Sunscreen You Should Never Use

Neal B. Schultz, MD, is an assistant clinical professor of dermatology at Mount Sinai's Icahn School of Medicine and runs his own practice, both in New York City. He also is the founder of *DermTV.com* and author of *It's Not Just About Wrinkles. NealSchultzMD.com*

Afraid to look in the mirror because it seems like Zorro is staring back? That mask-shaped pattern of darkened splotches on your forehead and below your eyes is called melasma. Though often referred to as the mask of pregnancy, melasma actually can develop at any time. Because it is linked to estrogen, the condition affects women about nine times more often than men...and it is particularly common among women who use hormone therapy, take birth control pills, or are or have been pregnant.

Melasma is very difficult to treat, so prevention is definitely the best approach. Since sun exposure triggers melasma, you'd think that sunscreen use would be the answer. And it is—but only if you use the right kind of sunscreen.

Here's why: Typical carbon-based sunscreens work by absorbing the sun's ultraviolet (UV) rays...and this chemical reaction generates enough heat to injure the hypersensitive pigment-producing cells in melasma-prone skin, causing even more dark blotches to appear!

Better: The so-called "chem-free" sun-protection products, which contain zinc oxide and/or titanium dioxide, are most appropriate for women with a history of melasma, said Neal B. Schultz, MD, an assistant clinical professor of dermatology at Mount Sinai School of Medicine and author of *It's Not Just About Wrinkles.* These products are not carbon-based, so they do not absorb UV rays—instead, they work by blocking or reflecting rays, as a mirror would.

Bottom line: The term "chem-free" may not appear on product labels. So to get the right sunscreen for your melasma-prone skin, look at the active ingredients list on the label to be sure that the product's only active ingredients are zinc oxide and/or titanium dioxide. Just a pea-sized dab will take care of your whole face.

How to Look 10 Years Younger in 1.3 Seconds

Laurie Steelsmith, ND, is the author of *Natural Choices for Women's Health* and a medical reviewer for Healthy-Woman from Bottom Line. Her private practice in naturopathic and Chinese medicine is in Honolulu. *Natural ChoicesForWomen.com*

Yes, you can look a little (or a lot) younger—and you can do it without much effort, expense or Real Housewives-like scary plastic surgery. Honolulu-based naturopathic physician Laurie Steelsmith, ND, author of *Natural Choices for Women's Health,* offers here an abundance of creative suggestions. Some take just minutes, others take almost no time at all...yet they can take as much as 10 years off a woman's appearance.

Youth-restoring options for when you have only 1.3 seconds to spare...

• **Project your "love glow."** A recent study from Syracuse University shows that falling in love takes only one-fifth of a second! Remember how new love could light you up from the inside, projecting youth and vitality? OK, maybe it's not possible to fall in love just now. But you can think a loving thought and give a big smile, Dr. Steelsmith said, which will bring a youthful sparkle to your face.

•**Check your posture.** Nothing reads old like slumping. For an instantly improved figure, stand up straight, raise your chin, throw those shoulders back and pull in your tummy.

•**Do a facial exercise.** Open your mouth and eyes wide…then scrunch up your face…then release. This gets the blood flowing, putting roses in your cheeks.

•**Brighten your eyes.** Use two drops of homeopathic Similasan eyedrops in each eye every three hours, as needed. This remedy, which is generally safe for everyone, reduces redness and soothes dryness and irritation, Dr. Steelsmith noted.

•**De-stress with instant aromatherapy.** The scent of lavender makes you feel—and look—more relaxed and rejuvenated. Lightly spritz yourself with a lavender product designed for use on the skin, such as Aura Cacia Lavender Harvest Aromatherapy Mist ($7.99 for four ounces at *www.AuraCacia.com*)…or rub a drop of lavender essential oil onto the pulse point on your wrist…or swirl four drops of lavender oil into your bathwater.

•**Dash on the right lipstick—a light-colored one.** Dark lipstick seems old-ladyish and actually emphasizes tiny lip lines.

•**Take a pass on heavy makeup.** Pancake foundation and too-bright blush look unnatural and make wrinkles more noticeable.

What to try when you have three minutes…

•**Exfoliate your face.** Getting rid of dead cells with a facial scrub makes your complexion glow. *Natural option:* Combine a spoonful of ground oatmeal with enough honey to make a paste, then gently rub it onto your clean face. Rinse.

•**Use contrast hydrotherapy.** To rinse your face, use two splashes of medium-hot water followed by two splashes of cold water. The hot/cold contrast increases circulation and tones skin, Dr. Steelsmith explained. *Next:* Moisten a cotton ball with a natural astringent, such as rose water, aloe vera juice or green tea, and stroke it across your face to remove lingering residue and restore the skin's proper pH.

•**Combat sun damage.** Smooth a dab of vitamin C serum over your face—its antioxidants protect against ultraviolet rays and environmental toxins. Dr. Steelsmith recommended the brands Obagi (*www.Obagi.com*) and SkinCeuticals (*www.SkinCeuticals.com*).

•**Counteract saggy eyelids.** Curling your eyelashes is a simple beauty technique that makes eyes appear larger.

•**Eat some blueberries.** Berries won't restore youthful comeliness instantly, of course—but they take just a moment to eat, and their vitamin C and bioflavanoids promote skin health and strengthen connective tissues.

If you can indulge yourself for 10 minutes…

•**Make your hair shine.** Rosemary essential oil gives tresses an extra sheen and a scent that's light and clean. It is particularly helpful for dry, brittle or frizzy hair. *After shampooing:* Add a few drops of rosemary oil to your conditioner, work through your hair for a few minutes, then rinse…or towel-dry your hair, rub a dab of rosemary oil between your palms and stroke it onto your damp hair. Then style as usual. Repeat after each shampoo (as Dr. Steelsmith does to keep her long hair frizz-free despite the Hawaiian humidity) or as often as desired.

•**Clear up blemishes.** Even if pimples remind you of being a teen, they don't make you look any younger. *The fix:* Use your fingertips to spread honey over your face, avoiding the eye area. Leave on for five minutes…rinse off with water…then cleanse your face as usual. "For people prone to acne, this works like a charm if used every day," Dr. Steelsmith said.

•**Give yourself a steam facial.** Steam cleans pores, boosts circulation and promotes a rosy complexion. *Dr. Steelsmith's method:* Fill a sink or bowl with steaming hot water. If desired, add a few drops of stimulating peppermint essential oil and/or anti-inflammatory lavender essential oil. Drape a towel over your head to trap the steam. Then bend over the water for several minutes, keeping eyes closed and taking care not to burn yourself.

•**Ease eye puffiness.** Dampen cotton balls with diluted witch hazel, then lie down with eyes closed and place the cotton balls over your eyes for five minutes (be careful not to let the witch hazel get into your eyes). Witch hazel contains catechol tannin, which reduces puffiness by constricting tiny capillaries just below the skin's surface.

●**Do some quickie aerobics.** Just 10 minutes of dancing or brisk walking increases circulation and reduces puffiness in the face, hands, ankles and elsewhere.

●**Drink a cleansing shake.** "I put many of my patients on a 'magic smoothie.' It is chock-full of vital nutrients and supports regular elimination, promoting the health and vitality of the whole body. And the healthier you are, the more youthful you tend to look," said Dr. Steelsmith. *To prepare two servings:* In a blender, combine one cup of chopped parsley or spinach…one chopped carrot…one-half chopped, peeled cucumber…one-half chopped, peeled apple…one banana…one-half cup blueberries…one heaping tablespoon of whey or rice protein powder…and two cups of water. Blend well. Enjoy immediately or refrigerate and drink later in the day.

Natural Ways to Younger-Looking Skin

Eudene Harry, MD, medical director of Oasis for Optimal Health in Orlando, Florida. She is the author of *Live Younger in 8 Simple Steps: A Practical Guide to Slowing Down the Aging Process from the Inside Out.* *LivingHealthyLookingYounger.com*

It's a fact of life that our skin becomes more wrinkled as we age. But you may be surprised to learn that our skin starts changing as early as age 30 for both women and men.

What happens: The cells that make up the skin divide more slowly with age, so the top layer of skin gets about 10% thinner every decade. The result? You guessed it—more wrinkles as well as more bruises…uneven skin tone…and sagging skin. Of course, you can "refresh" your appearance with Botox and skin fillers, but even "inexpensive" cosmetic procedures cost hundreds of dollars.

A better option: Natural skin care. Used properly, natural approaches can take years off your appearance.

STEP 1: TWEAK YOUR DIET

While you might think that skin-care products are the logical choice to smooth wrinkled skin, it's wise to first work from the "inside out" to give your skin the nutrients it needs to look its best.

Increasing laboratory evidence and positive reports from patients suggest that the following foods promote younger-looking skin…

●**High-sulfur foods.** Sulfur is known to be one of the "building blocks" of collagen, a protein that strengthens skin and gives it elasticity. Fortunately, sulfur is found in a number of foods.

My advice: At least once a day, eat sulfur-rich foods.

Good choices: Eggs, chives, legumes (such as black, white or kidney beans) and fish that is high in omega-3 fatty acids (such as salmon and sardines).

●**Grape juice or red wine.** These contain flavonoids known as proanthocyanidins and proteins called tenascins—both help make the skin smoother and more elastic.

My advice: Enjoy a daily glass of grape juice—or red wine if your doctor says daily alcohol consumption is appropriate for you. Both are high in proanthocyanidins.

In addition, a grape seed extract supplement (typical dose 200 mg once a day) is beneficial, but check first with your doctor if you take medication, especially a blood thinner—the supplement may interact with certain drugs.

●**Soy foods.** Tofu, soy milk and other foods derived from soy can make skin appear significantly younger. This is mainly due to genistein, an antioxidant in soy that slows skin aging and increases collagen. Genistein and other compounds are linked to increased skin elasticity and plumpness. These compounds give the skin a "glow" that makes it appear younger.

My advice: Have one or more daily servings of soy foods.

Good choices: Edamame (steamed soy beans) and miso (a fermented paste used in cooking). Check first with your doctor if you have breast cancer or kidney disease or take any medication. Soy may be harmful for some breast cancer and kidney disease patients...it may also interact with certain drugs, including blood thinners and some antidepressants.

Also: To help keep skin hydrated, drink eight eight-ounce glasses of water each day.

STEP 2: USE THE RIGHT SKIN-CARE PRODUCTS

Skin-care products can help smooth wrinkles and provide other benefits, but there are so many on the market that most people are confused about which to use. *Best choices for younger-looking skin...*

•**Topical vitamin C.** About 80% of the dermis (the second layer of skin) consists of that all important protein collagen. Because collagen production declines with age, it's a good idea to promote collagen production any way you can.

That's where vitamin C enters the picture. The body uses vitamin C to produce collagen, but whatever is consumed orally doesn't reach adequate concentrations in the skin to boost collagen. That's why you need to apply it topically.

My advice: Use skin-care products (such as lotions and sunscreens) that have ascorbic acid (vitamin C)—the best form of the vitamin for absorption as well as collagen production and sun protection. Studies show that topical vitamin C can reduce the appearance of fine lines and wrinkles in as little as three months.

To save money: Buy powdered vitamin C at a health-food store, and mix in a small pinch each time you use a moisturizer/sunscreen that does not contain the vitamin.

•**Retinoic acid.** This is a form of vitamin A that is added to hundreds of over-the-counter (OTC) skin-care products. It is also available by prescription. Retinoic acid increases cellular turnover, the rate at which cells divide.

This makes the skin appear brighter, smoother and plumper.

My advice: Use OTC retinol cream once daily. Apply it at night because it temporarily increases the skin's sensitivity to sun. Most products have a concentration of 1% or less. Prescription-strength retinoic acid usually is not necessary.

•**Moisturizer.** Everyone should use this as they age. Adding moisture to skin cells makes them expand, which improves skin volume and texture. Moisturizers protect the skin from environmental factors (heat, dryness and pollution) that undermine skin health.

My advice: Use moisturizer with sunscreen at least twice a day. I advise a vitamin C–enhanced moisturizer that includes green-tea extract. Both ingredients improve the skin's ability to absorb the moisturizer. Compounds in green tea also reduce skin inflammation and sun-related skin damage. Soy moisturizers may provide similar benefits.

Also important: Exfoliation, an effective form of controlled trauma that stimulates the skin to produce more collagen. Every week or two, use a gentle facial scrub with fine grains and a soft facial brush. This practice also removes the dead skin cells that dull your complexion.

Sensitive skin sometimes cannot tolerate even a mild scrub. An ultrasonic brush, such as Clarisonic ($100 to $200 at department stores and online), with a hydrating cleanser is a good alternative.

A chemical peel once or twice a year is another good way to remove dead skin cells. OTC peels contain glycolic acid, lactic acid or salicylic acid, usually in a concentration of about 5% to 10%. Peels should also contain moisturizing ingredients to minimize irritation. If you're new to chemical peels, talk with your dermatologist before using one of these products, since they can irritate skin, especially sensitive skin.

Home Remedies for Softer, Smoother Hands

Laurie Steelsmith, ND, LAc, is the author of *Natural Choices for Women's Health* and coauthor with Alex Steelsmith of the upcoming *Great Sex Naturally* (Hay House). Her private practice in naturopathic and Chinese medicine is in Honolulu. *NaturalChoicesForWomen.com*

No matter what time of year it is, hands can easily become dry and scaly. With all these brand-name products available, it's easy to get confused…especially since many commercial products have unwanted ingredients.

For instance: Alcohol, which can leave skin even more parched…mineral oil, which can clog pores…preservatives, which can dry and damage skin…and/or a high water content, which makes the products less emollient and thus less able to penetrate and hydrate the skin.

Laurie Steelsmith, ND, a naturopathic physician in Honolulu and author of *Natural Choices for Women's Health,* has advice. Here she shares four simple recipes for hand-healing remedies. Each can be made at home with inexpensive, all-natural ingredients you already have or can easily find at the health-food store. Use any or all of the following remedies as often as you like.

For dry, dehydrated hands: Milk Soak. In a medium-size glass bowl, heat two cups of whole milk in the microwave until pleasantly warm to the touch—do not overheat. Soak your hands in the milk for five to 10 minutes, then rinse hands well. Dr. Steelsmith explained that milk (especially whole milk) contains fats that moisturize and hydrate the skin…plus calcium, vitamin A and vitamin E that nourish the skin cells (nails, too).

For scaly, flaky hands: Oatmeal-Sea Salt Scrub. In a small bowl, sift one cup of instant oats (which are finer than steel-cut or rolled oats) between your fingers, removing any sharp hulls. Mix in one tablespoon of finely ground sea salt. Stir in one to two tablespoons of whole milk, a bit at a time, until the mixture is moist and sticky. Rub the oats mixture all over your hands, massaging it in for several minutes—this acts as an exfoliant to remove dead skin cells. Rinse hands well.

For irritated or itchy hands: Nighttime Nourisher. In a small bowl, combine two tablespoons of olive oil, two drops of calendula extract and two drops of chamomile extract. At bedtime, rub the oil mixture into your hands for several minutes, then put on cotton gloves and leave on overnight. In the morning, remove gloves and wash hands with gentle soap. Olive oil is a natural nonirritating moisturizer…and calendula and chamomile have healing properties that soothe sensitive skin, Dr. Steelsmith explained.

For multiple hand woes: All-in-One Honey Treatment. In a bowl, combine one-quarter cup of lard, one egg yolk, one-half tablespoon of honey, one-half tablespoon of ground almonds and a few drops of rosewater for scent. Massage the mixture into your hands, then leave it on until it hardens, about 15 to 30 minutes. Wash off with warm water and a gentle soap. Although this treatment requires more ingredients than the other remedies, Dr. Steelsmith said that its many benefits—moisturizing, nourishing, exfoliating, healing—make it worth the effort when you need extra help.

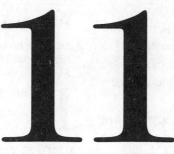

11

Help for Vaginal Infections and More

Soothing Healer for Vaginal Infections

Those unwelcome, yet all too familiar, signs—vaginal itching and burning, icky discharge, nasty odor—announce that a vaginal bacterial or yeast infection has made an appearance. Can you fight back without resorting to antibiotics or antifungal medication? Yes, you can, with *Lactobacillus acidophilus* vaginal suppositories, says Laurie Steelsmith, ND, author of *Natural Choices for Women's Health*.

Unhealthful bacteria and fungi thrive when the pH of the vagina becomes too alkaline, she explained. Using Lactobacillus suppositories, starting as soon as symptoms appear, populates the vagina with friendly bacteria, which in turn restores a healthy, more acidic vaginal pH. This combats existing infections…and ultimately helps prevent future infections.

Lactobacillus vaginal suppositories are sold in health-food stores and online. Dr. Steelsmith

recommended Gy-Na-Tren Vaginal Health Kit ($27 at *www.natren.com*), which is used daily for up to two weeks. The kit has two separate products—14 vaginal suppositories of a specific and effective strain of Lactobacillus combined with homeopathic Boricum acidum…plus 14 oral Lactobacillus pills to further support vaginal health.

A more economical alternative is to make your own suppositories using plain, sugar-free yogurt and the o.b. brand of tampon (which has no applicator and is inserted with a finger). Dr. Steelsmith advised, "Coat the outside of the tampon with yogurt—don't soak it or it will get too wet—then quickly insert it into the vagina and leave it there for one hour. Do this once daily until symptoms are gone, then stop. Typically, this takes as few as three treatments, but intractable cases of bacterial vaginosis or

Laurie Steelsmith, ND, LAc, is the author of *Natural Choices for Women's Health* and coauthor with Alex Steelsmith of the upcoming *Great Sex Naturally*. Her private practice in naturopathic and Chinese medicine is in Honolulu. *NaturalChoicesForWomen.com* chronic unrelenting yeast infections may take up to 14 days of treatments to be completely resolved. I also recommend using these suppositories to prevent a vaginal yeast infection whenever you are taking oral antibiotics." Do not continue indefinitely—overuse can cause an overgrowth of Lactobacillus that exacerbates itching.

With either method, if your symptoms are not completely resolved within two weeks, see your doctor. You may have a different condition, such as a sexually transmitted disease, that will not respond to Lactobacillus suppositories.

What to Do with Vaginal Itch

Many people assume that the culprit in vaginal itching is a yeast infection—but this is not necessarily so. Your problem could be a sensitivity to chemical irritants in perfumed laundry detergents, fabric softeners, dryer sheets or soaps...so try fragrance-free products.

Another possible cause is pubic-hair shaving or waxing. Pubic hair serves a purpose—it absorbs potentially irritating moisture and protects the skin of the outer vaginal area.

Best: Let the hair grow naturally, or trim minimally.

Also, wear 100% cotton panties. True, nylon panties look sexier—but nylon can cause itching by trapping moisture. Even when nylon panties have a cotton crotch sewn inside, moisture can be a problem unless you cut off the nylon that covers the cotton on the outside...which ends up looking not-so-sexy.

Cherie A. LeFevre, MD, associate professor, division of gynecologic sub-specialties, and staff at the Vulvar and Vaginal Disorders Specialty Center, Saint Louis University School of Medicine, St. Louis.

Treating a UTI Without Antibiotics

Sergei Frenzel, ND, MD, is the founder of Integrative Natural Health, a clinic in Milford, Connecticut.

Is there any way to get rid of recurrent urinary tract infections without taking antibiotics? One good approach is to increase your urine flow, which helps by pushing harmful bacteria out of the urinary tract, giving them less time to multiply. To achieve this, boost your fluid intake. You should be drinking about two quarts (eight cups) of water per day when healthy, so try increasing this—up to four quarts per day if you can—when you have a urinary tract infection (UTI).

Second, you want to adjust your urine's pH (a measure of acidity or alkalinity). The types of bacteria that cause UTIs tend to thrive in a more alkaline environment, so the goal is to make your urine more acidic. Taking 1,000 mg of vitamin C every four to six hours during a UTI helps move urine pH in the right direction. Drinking unsweetened cranberry juice or taking cranberry capsules also makes urine more acidic.

Third, you can supplement with herbs that have antibacterial qualities, such as echinacea, hydrastis (goldenseal) and/or uva ursi (bearberry). Herbal teas and tinctures are sold in health-food stores...or you can use a combination herbal product designed to improve urinary tract health, such as Wise Woman Herbals Urinary Tract Formula Liquid Extract Compound (*www.wisewomanherbals.com*).

See your doctor if you are not feeling better within several days or if you experience any worsening of UTI symptoms (such as increased urinary discomfort, fever or back pain). At that point, you may need antibiotics or you may benefit from a more individualized approach to UTI treatment.

Probiotics for Vaginal Health

Laurie Cullen, ND, chair of the department of clinical sciences and faculty in the School of Naturopathic Medicine, Bastyr University, Kenmore, Washington, and core clinical faculty member, Bastyr Center for Natural Health, Seattle.

You know how helpful probiotics are for your digestive health…but did you know that these beneficial bacteria also promote vaginal health?

Folk medicine has long recommended eating yogurt as a natural remedy for vaginal infections, and now studies are finding evidence that folk wisdom was on the right track. For instance, a recent study in *Journal of Family Practice* showed that the probiotics in yogurt and in certain vaginal suppositories may reduce the recurrence of bacterial vaginosis (BV), the most common type of vaginal infection among women of childbearing age.

Although we don't yet have a large body of peer-reviewed research proving that probiotics prevent various types of recurrent vaginal infections, it just makes sense to use beneficial bacteria to battle harmful bacteria, said Laurie Cullen, ND, chair, clinical sciences and faculty in the School of Naturopathic Medicine at Bastyr University, whose practice focuses on women's health.

"The vaginal ecosystem is very sensitive," Dr. Cullen explained. "The beneficial Lactobacilli strains of bacteria that live in the vagina keep the pH around 4.2. Certain factors can raise the vaginal pH, leading to an overgrowth of various bacteria and causing BV. Situations that lower the vaginal pH can lead to an overgrowth of fungal organisms, such as Candida albicans, and cause a yeast infection."

Among the many factors that can affect vaginal pH are the use of antibiotics, oral steroid medications, spermicidal contraceptives or birth control pills…sexual intercourse, menstruation, tampon use, pregnancy or menopause…diabetes or obesity…cancer or cancer treatment…and conditions that compromise the immune system.

PROBIOTICS FOR PREVENTION

The following prevention strategies are appropriate for just about any woman who wants to keep her vagina as healthy as possible…and they're particularly helpful for those who have a history of vaginal infections.

Note: Whatever type of probiotic you use—be it in the form of yogurt, an oral supplement or a topical vaginal product—avoid brands that contain only the species of Lactobacillus called acidophilus. "Acidophilus, which comes from cow's milk, is really good at populating a cow's vagina with cow-beneficial probiotics, but on its own it doesn't do much to help repopulate the human vagina with the various Lactobacilli species normally found there," Dr. Cullen explained. She recommends probiotics that contain a number of different Lactobacillus species in addition to acidophilus, such as Lactobacillus GG, rhamnosus, reuteri, plantarum and/or salvarius.

Dr. Cullen suggested trying one, two or all three of the types of products below for two to six months to see if they help your vagina stay infection-free. If so, you can continue to use them indefinitely.

● **Cultured yogurt.** Eat at least one serving daily. For women who like dairy yogurt, Dr. Cullen recommended the plain-flavored Stonyfield brand. For people who prefer a cultured soymilk yogurt alternative, she suggested the Silk brand's Fruity & Creamy line. Why does she like these brands? "Because we can verify the cultures, meaning that we can grow in a lab the bacteria that they say are in their product," she explained.

● **Oral probiotics.** For her patients, Dr. Cullen most often prescribes over-the-counter oral supplements such as FemDophilus…FemEcology…or Pro-Flora Women's Probiotic by Integrative Therapeutics. Usually these are taken daily, following the guidelines on the product label.

● **Vaginal moisturizers.** Sex affects the vaginal pH because men's semen has a pH of about 7.1 to 8.0. Spermicidal contraceptives also alter the pH of the vagina. A vaginal moisturizer helps keep the vaginal pH in balance, which is why it's a good idea to use one before and immediately after having sex. Also use it daily whenever you are taking antibiotics. Dr.

Cullen's preferred brands include RepHresh Vaginal Gel…and Luvena Restorative Vaginal Moisturizer.

TREATING GYNO CONDITIONS WITH PROBIOTICS

If you develop any symptoms of a vaginal infection, such as itching, discharge, odor and/or pain, it's important to see a doctor who can diagnose the cause. "Women who try self-treatment without first getting a diagnosis may end up making the problem worse," Dr. Cullen cautioned. Treatment depends on the type of infection your doctor ends up diagnosing. *The most common types are…*

•**Yeast vaginitis.** For her patients with vaginal yeast infections, Dr. Cullen relies on vaginal suppositories of boric acid (also called borax). Although such suppositories are available without a prescription, before using them, you should make sure that your doctor confirms the yeast diagnosis. If you are prone to recurrent yeast infections and your doctor is satisfied that you can recognize the symptoms, however, he/she may give you the go-ahead to self-treat. In such cases, Dr. Cullen often prescribes a five-to-seven-day course of Yeast Arrest Suppositories, which contain several homeopathic anti-yeast ingredients in addition to boric acid.

After the boric acid treatment is done, Dr. Cullen said, it's a good idea to help restore vaginal health by inserting a probiotic product directly into the vagina once daily for one to two weeks. For this, Dr. Cullen recommends capsules of FemDophilus, FemEcology or Pro-Flora Women's Probiotic—yes, the same oral probiotic supplements mentioned in the prevention section above also can be used as vaginal suppositories, she said.

•**Bacterial vaginosis.** For her patients with BV, Dr. Cullen typically recommends using FemDophilus, FemEcology or Pro-Flora Women's Probiotic both orally and vaginally—one oral and one vaginal capsule per day. Sometimes this strategy provides enough immune support to allow a woman's body to fight off the infection. However, if this approach doesn't work within three or four days, it may be necessary to use antibiotics to get rid of BV.

Thumbs Up or Down For Thongs?

Paul Nyirjesy, MD, is a professor of obstetrics and gynecology at Drexel University College of Medicine and director of the Drexel Vaginitis Center, both in Philadelphia. He has been listed among *Philadelphia* magazine's Top Doctors numerous times.

Have you read those Internet articles about the potential health threats of thong underwear? You know, the ones likening that thin strip of fabric to a bacterial conveyor belt—sliding back and forth between the buttocks, carrying fecal matter forward and triggering recurrent vaginal and/or urinary tract infections. If so, perhaps you said, "So long, thongs"…or perhaps, unwilling to accept visible panty lines, you still wear thongs at times but feel anxious or unhygienic when you do. Either way, the question is this: Just how credible are those reports?

The answer comes from Paul Nyirjesy, MD, a professor of obstetrics and gynecology at Drexel University College of Medicine and director of the Drexel Vaginitis Center, both in Philadelphia. "Women who like this type of underwear can breathe a sigh of relief because there is nothing unhygienic about wearing thongs. No studies have shown any increase in infections from bacteria spreading from the anus to the vagina or urethra, nor is there evidence of any increased risk for yeast infections," he said.

One thing you should watch out for, however, is excessive tightness. Thongs, by design, tend to fit rather snugly. But no matter what style of undies you wear—thongs, G-strings, bikinis, briefs, boxers—a pair that is tight enough to leave marks anywhere on your skin also might be tight enough to irritate and inflame delicate anal and vulvar tissues. This could lead to itching, pain and an increased susceptibility to infection, Dr. Nyirjesy cautioned.

Bottom line: No need to worry. If you like 'em, wear 'em.

Perfect Fabrics
For Panties

Paul Nyirjesy, MD, is a professor of obstetrics and gynecology at Drexel University College of Medicine and director of the Drexel Vaginitis Center, both in Philadelphia. He has been listed among *Philadelphia* magazine's Top Doctors numerous times.

Cherie A. LeFevre, MD, associate professor, division of gynecologic sub-specialties, and staff at the Vulvar and Vaginal Disorders Specialty Center, Saint Louis University School of Medicine, St. Louis.

Which type of panty fabric is best for genital health? This is a very good question with surprisingly little scientific data to address it, considering the vast array of panty choices available at stores. Still, many vaginal health experts agree that cotton generally is superior for everyday wear. Cotton panties are nonirritating and create no friction that could irritate vulvar tissues. Silk, satin and spandex are OK, provided they have a cotton crotch.

When you are exercising or if you tend to sweat a lot, consider a moisture-wicking synthetic fabric or cotton/polyester blend. Excess wetness and heat in the vulvar area can create a breeding ground for bacteria and yeast, increasing your risk for vaginal infections. Whenever your panties do feel damp, switch to a fresh pair as soon as possible.

Avoid panties made completely of nylon, as this fabric restricts airflow and traps moisture. Also steer clear of panties that have scratchy or abrasive lace or seams at the crotch. As a further safeguard against vulvar irritation, when laundering panties, avoid detergents, fabric softeners and dryer sheets—instead, stick with a mild enzyme-free soap (such as Woolite or All Free Clear), using only one-half to one-third the suggested amount.

Protect Yourself from
Pedicure Infections

Skin infections from spa pedicures are becoming common.

Self-defense: Broken skin should not come in contact with foot-bath water. Don't shave, wax or use hair-removal cream on legs in the 24 hours before going to a foot spa. Don't go to the spa if you have skin damage, such as cuts or bug bites, on your feet or lower-leg area. Ask salon workers if foot spas are disinfected after each customer and again at night with a hospital disinfectant.

Recommendations from the US Environmental Protection Agency.

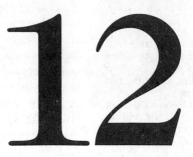

PMS and Menopause Relief

Natural Help for Painful Periods

I'm frequently asked by patients—either for themselves or on behalf of family members—about natural treatments for menstrual cramps. Cramping, which is characterized by inflammation, is caused by high levels of certain prostaglandins that trigger uterine contractions. Often high prostaglandin levels are accompanied by estrogen dominance, where estrogen levels are too high relative to progesterone. Using specific nutrients, I am able to balance the ratio between these hormones in patients and greatly relieve cramping.

You can use just one of the remedies below or all of them, depending on what helps you. You need to take most of these remedies all month (as indicated), even though symptoms occur on only a few days, because these remedies don't just treat symptoms. Instead, they work to enhance the release of progesterone…improve circulation…or relax muscles.

• **Vitex.** This herb (also known as chasteberry) improves the production of progesterone and offsets estrogen dominance.

Dose: 160 mg to 240 mg, or 40 drops of tincture daily. Try it for at least three months. If it helps you, you can keep taking it. Don't use vitex if you are taking birth control pills.

• **Pycnogenol.** This pine bark extract contains potent anti-inflammatories and antioxidants. It boosts production of endothelial nitric oxide, which improves circulation and helps to reduce the pain of cramps. A Japanese study found that pycnogenol significantly decreased the amount of time women had menstrual cramps.

Dose: 100 mg to 150 mg daily.

Mark A. Stengler, NMD, is a naturopathic medical doctor and leading authority on the practice of alternative and integrated medicine. Dr. Stengler is author of the *Health Revelations* newsletter, author of *The Natural Physician's Healing Therapies,* founder and medical director of the Stengler Center for Integrative Medicine in Encinitas, California, and adjunct associate clinical professor at the National College of Natural Medicine in Portland, Oregon. *MarkStengler.com*

•**Calcium and magnesium.** These minerals reduce premenstrual syndrome symptoms. Magnesium acts as a muscle relaxant, relieving cramps.

Dose: A daily calcium supplement of 500 mg to 1,000 mg that contains at least half as much magnesium. It may take one to two menstrual cycles to reduce symptoms.

•**Natural progesterone.** For severe menstrual cramps, I recommend bioidentical progesterone cream to reduce estrogen dominance. A typical dose is 20 mg twice daily starting two weeks before menses. Work with a holistic physician who can monitor your hormone levels while you use it.

Feeling Anxious? Passionflower Can Calm You Down

Mark A. Stengler, NMD, is a naturopathic medical doctor and leading authority on the practice of alternative and integrated medicine. Dr. Stengler is author of the *Health Revelations* newsletter, author of *The Natural Physician's Healing Therapies*, founder and medical director of the Stengler Center for Integrative Medicine in Encinitas, California, and adjunct associate clinical professor at the National College of Natural Medicine in Portland, Oregon. *MarkStengler.com*

Its name suggests an aphrodisiac, but passionflower is more effective for relaxation than arousal. The herb increases the brain's levels of gamma-amino-butyric acid (GABA), which helps people relax. It is available at health-food stores and online. *How it can help…*

•**Insomnia.** Australian researchers found that adults who drank a warm herbal infusion of passionflower before bed felt refreshed and alert upon waking, compared with those drinking a placebo tea.

•**Anxiety.** Passionflower can help you relax without causing drowsiness, which makes it particularly good as a daytime remedy. How can a remedy that helps you sleep also enable you to stay awake? That's one of the great things about passionflower—it enhances (instead of works against) the body's natural sleep/wake cycle.

•**PMS and menopause.** Passionflower can help to relieve PMS symptoms and menopausal symptoms of anxiety and irritability.

•**High blood pressure.** Passionflower is known to reduce high blood pressure associated with stress and anxiety.

How to use it: For patients who want relief from the conditions above, I recommend passionflower be taken in capsule form (500 milligrams) two to three times daily when symptoms occur. It also can be taken as a tincture (20 to 30 drops) or herbal infusion (one teaspoon of dried passionflower leaves steeped in three ounces of water) taken two to three times daily. Women who are pregnant should not use passionflower. It should not be taken with pharmaceutical sedatives because it may increase their effect.

Natural Ways to Ease Menopause Symptoms

Ann Louise Gittleman, PhD, nutritionist based in Post Falls, Idaho, and author of more than 30 books, including *Hot Times: How to Eat Well, Live Healthy, and Feel Sexy During the Change.*

For decades, women relied on hormone replacement therapy (HRT) to relieve symptoms of menopause—hot flashes, sleep disturbance, anxiety and mood swings. But several large studies have linked long-term HRT with increased risk of breast cancer, dementia, heart attack and stroke.

Fortunately, there are safer, natural alternatives to HRT.

MORE THAN JUST ESTROGEN

People typically attribute menopausal symptoms to declining production of the female hormones estrogen and progesterone. But poor eating and lifestyle habits also play a role, by overtaxing the adrenal glands. For women who are going through menopause, the adrenal glands are nature's backup system. When the ovaries decrease their production of estrogen and progesterone, the adrenals have the ability to produce hormones to compensate. Poor diet and lifestyle choices put stress on the adrenals, creating an imbalance in body chemistry and contributing to the uncomfortable symptoms that we associate with menopause.

If you are a woman with menopausal symptoms, adopting healthier habits can help to even out these imbalances.

If you are a man and the woman you love is going through menopause, you can help by understanding that she is experiencing a profound physiological change. Your kindness and patience can ease her transition through a time that is confusing—for her as well as for you.

Common symptoms and natural solutions...

HOT FLASHES

As many as 80% of women experience hot flashes during menopause. One theory is that the hypothalamus, which controls body temperature, is triggered in some way by hormonal fluctuations.

•**Avoid spicy foods.** Foods containing cayenne or other peppers have a thermogenic effect, meaning that they raise body temperature.

•**Cook with garlic, onion, thyme, oregano and sage.** These seasonings contain very small amounts of phytoestrogens (plant-based estrogens such as lignans and isoflavones that occur naturally in certain foods) and can help restore hormone balance.

•**Cut down on caffeine.** Caffeine stimulates the adrenal glands, leading to a spike in blood sugar levels followed by a plunge in blood sugar to even lower levels than before. This stresses the body and aggravates menopause woes.

If you don't want to give up coffee completely, have one cup a day with food. Don't use coffee as a stimulant between meals. Instead, eat frequent small meals for energy.

Better than coffee: Green, white and black teas have less caffeine and are high in disease-fighting antioxidants. Try substituting tea for coffee. Then transition to herbal tea or hot water with lemon.

•**Add flaxseed.** Ground flaxseed contains lignans, which seem to modulate fluctuating estrogen and progesterone levels. Aim for two tablespoons a day. Ground flaxseed has a pleasant nutty flavor—sprinkle it on cereal, yogurt and salads.

Bonus: Flaxseed reduces cholesterol, helps prevent certain cancers and relieves constipation (be sure to drink plenty of water).

•**Eat soy foods in moderation.** Some countries with diets high in soy report low rates of menopausal symptoms and breast cancer. But I'm cautious about soy. Preliminary research suggests that while isoflavones in soy appear to protect against some breast cancers, they may stimulate growth of other types of breast cancer.

I'm especially concerned about isolated soy protein, which often is added to protein powder, energy bars and supplements. This puts far more soy isoflavones into the diet than other cultures typically consume—and these high amounts may not be healthful.

If you enjoy soy foods, limit your consumption to two servings a week, and eat them in their whole-food form—as tofu, tempeh, miso and edamame.

•**Be wary of herbal remedies.** I'm cautious about black cohosh, red clover and other plant remedies with estrogenlike properties. Research has not demonstrated clearly that they help, and some can have harmful side effects if not properly monitored. However, some women do report good results from these remedies. Check with your doctor first. If you don't notice a clear change in symptoms after two to three weeks of trying a new remedy, ask your doctor about trying something else.

What men can do: Buy a dual-control electric blanket so that you both will be comfortable. Make her a cup of herbal tea. Join her in eating flaxseed—it is good for your colon and prostate.

INSOMNIA

During menopause, elevated levels of the stress hormone cortisol make it difficult to fall asleep and can trigger intermittent awakening throughout the night. *Natural sleep aids...*

•**Wild yam cream.** This topical cream extracted from yams grown in Mexico is a source of natural progesterone. It's available at most health-food stores and some pharmacies. Applying small amounts of wild yam cream daily may help to balance cortisol levels and enhance sleep. (The cream also helps reduce anxiety and hot flashes.)

Apply one-quarter teaspoon once in the morning and once at night. Gently rub the cream into areas where you see capillaries, such as the wrist, back of the knee and neck—these are the places where skin is thinnest and the cream is easily absorbed. Alternate where you apply the cream on a daily basis.

•**Magnesium.** Levels of magnesium, a natural sleep aid, are depleted when you consume too much coffee, cola, alcohol, sugar or salt. Foods high in magnesium include halibut…whole-wheat bread…leafy green vegetables such as spinach…nuts…and dried beans (soaked and cooked). If your diet is low in magnesium, take 200 milligrams (mg) to 400 mg in supplement form at bedtime.

•**Zinc.** This mineral can help quiet an overactive mind. Foods rich in zinc include poultry, red meat and nuts, but it is hard to get enough zinc from food. Take 25 mg to 45 mg in supplement form before bed.

•**Exercise.** One study found that women over age 50 who walked, biked or did stretching exercises every morning fell asleep more easily. Try to get a half-hour of exercise most mornings. Avoid working out in the evening—you may have trouble winding down. And don't go to extremes. Overexercising (more than two hours of strenuous, nonstop activity every day) can lead to hormonal imbalance.

What men can do: Exercise with her in the morning. Make sure there is a bottle of magnesium tablets by the bedside at home and when traveling.

MOOD SWINGS

Drinking less coffee and eating frequent small meals will go a long way toward balancing your moods by reducing spikes in blood sugar and stress on adrenals. *In addition…*

•**Eat a balanced diet.** The emotional and mental stress of menopause can lead to a vicious cycle in which stress depletes important mineral stores, further taxing the adrenals.

Among the minerals depleted by stress are copper, calcium, magnesium, potassium, sodium and zinc. To restore these minerals, eat an adrenal-supportive diet rich in bright-colored fruits and vegetables, legumes, lean meats and whole grains. Avoid sugar and other refined carbohydrates.

Recommended: Sea vegetables, such as nori, arame, wakame and hijiki. These are especially high in key minerals. Health-food stores sell them in dried form. They can be crumbled into soup and over fish, salad and vegetables.

•**Get the right kind of fat.** Though you should avoid saturated fats (found in pork, beef and high-fat dairy products) and hydrogenated fats (in margarine, shortening and many packaged baked goods), certain fats are necessary for hormonal regulation and proper functioning of the nervous system. Known as essential fatty acids (EFAs), these healthy fats help to stabilize blood sugar.

Strive to consume two tablespoons a day of healthy oil (use it in cooking, salad dressings, etc.). Olive, sesame, almond, macadamia and flaxseed oils are especially high in EFAs. (Flaxseed oil does not cook well.)

•**Take B-complex vitamins.** B vitamins are known as the antistress vitamins because they nourish the adrenals. Good sources of B vitamins include whole grains and dried beans (soaked and cooked). Most diets are too low in these vitamins, so supplements usually are needed to make up the deficit. Take 50 mg to 100 mg of a vitamin-B complex daily.

What men can do: Make it easy for her to avoid sugar and caffeine by cutting back on them yourself—your health will benefit, too. If she seems distant or on edge, don't take it personally. Remind yourself that it is not you—it is her biochemistry that is acting up.

WEIGHT GAIN

One reason why so many women gain weight during menopause is that the ovulation process burns calories—as many as 300 per day during the first 10 days of the menstrual cycle. When ovulation stops, fewer calories are burned and metabolism slows. *Foods to counter the slowdown...*

●**Protein.** Increasing protein intake can raise the body's metabolic rate by as much as 25%. Aim for three to four ounces of lean protein from fish, poultry, beef or lamb twice a day. Eggs and beans also are good sources.

●**Healthy carbohydrates.** Whole grains, vegetables and fruits metabolize slowly and give you energy throughout the day. Try to consume daily at least two servings of fruits, three servings of vegetables and three servings of whole grains.

What men can do: Don't nag her about her weight. Support her by not buying high-calorie foods, such as potato chips and rich desserts.

Hot Flashes and High Blood Pressure

Linda M. Gerber, PhD, professor of healthcare policy and research, Weill Cornell Medical College in New York City.

Andrew L. Rubman, ND, director, Southbury Clinic for Traditional Medicines, Southbury, Connecticut.

Most of us women know that simply reaching midlife puts us at greater risk for heart disease, since we tend to lose the protective effects of estrogen. While previous research has linked menopause to high blood pressure (a major risk factor for heart attack), a new study links one of its most irksome symptoms—hot flashes—to high blood pressure. With hot flashes—defined as being sudden feelings of intense heat that may include sweating and a rapid heartbeat, and lasting usually from two to 30 minutes—being one of the major hallmarks of menopause and perimenopause, this study may be a "red alert" to identify a danger signal for women at risk of future heart problems.

Researchers at Weill Cornell Medical College in New York City found that women who had hot flashes tended to have higher systolic (top

number) blood pressure compared with the lucky ones who didn't have hot flashes. In the study, 154 women aged 18 to 65 with no previous cardiovascular disease and who either had normal blood pressure or mild hypertension (high blood pressure) wore portable monitors that recorded their blood pressure while they were awake and asleep. Women who reported having hot flashes were found to have an age-adjusted average systolic blood pressure of 141 while awake, and 129 while they were asleep, compared with 132 and 119, respectively, for women who did not report hot flashes. The blood pressure differences between these two groups remained statistically significant after controlling for high blood pressure risk factors including race/ethnicity, age and body mass index (BMI).

"One-third of the women we studied reported having had hot flashes two weeks prior to wearing a BP monitor," said Linda M. Gerber, PhD, the study's lead author, who is a professor of healthcare policy and research at Weill Cornell Medical College in New York City. "Among these women, systolic blood pressure was significantly higher—even after adjusting for whether they were pre-menopausal, menopausal or post-menopausal."

DO WOMEN WITH HOT FLASHES HAVE TO WORRY?

So if you are experiencing hot flashes, even only once in a while, should you worry that you may be at risk for high blood pressure? "You should keep your eye on it, but not be unduly concerned," said Dr. Gerber. "It's important to get an accurate representation of your blood pressure, but that is often difficult to get. Blood pressure varies over the course of the day. Some people get the white coat effect, in which your blood pressure is high when you go to see your doctor. I don't want people to rush to see their doctors. One way to keep an eye on it would be to get a home monitor and check it on a frequent basis."

And what about those pesky hot flashes? "You can do things that might be beneficial to limit the severity and frequency of your hot flashes," said Dr. Gerber. "Keep your weight down, exercise regularly and eat a healthy diet."

Andrew L. Rubman, ND, adds that the association between estrogen reduction and both hot flashes and increased systolic blood pressure may be due to concentrations of calcium within the tissue responsible for both. There are effective natural ways to modulate this, including black cohosh and soy isoflavones, but it's important to work with an experienced expert, such as a naturopathic physician, to ensure safety.

Most important, adds Dr. Gerber: "Be aware that if the frequency of hot flashes increases suddenly and if you have a lot of severe flashes when you didn't have them before, you should get your blood pressure checked."

New Map for the Menopause Maze

William F. Young, Jr., MD, MSc, chair, endocrinology, diabetes, metabolism and nutrition department, Mayo Clinic, Rochester, Minnesota and former president of The Endocrine Society, an international organization devoted to research on hormones and the clinical practice of endocrinology, based in Chevy Chase, Maryland.

Menopause is a nightmare," my friend Monica moaned. "When a hot flash hits, I feel like I'm in Hades. I wake up half a dozen times every night. And sex is so excruciating that I'm tempted to swear off it."

Sounds bad! Yet when I asked what treatment Monica was considering, she said that she hadn't bothered to bring up the subject with her doctor. Why not? Because she was too scared of the side effects to even consider taking hormones...she didn't think anything else could help...and it seemed to her that the whole topic was a confusing and contradictory maze of myths and misinformation.

Monica is typical. In fact, among women currently experiencing menopausal symptoms, more than 60% have not talked to their doctors about hormone therapy or nonhormone options, and 72% have not received any treatment for their symptoms, according to a survey from The Endocrine Society.

That's why I'm eager to tell you about a new online resource that can help you sort out your treatment options and provide talking points to discuss with your doctor. The free interactive Web tool, called the Menopause Map, can be accessed at *www.Hormone.org* (search "Menopause Map").

Relief Rx: Recently launched by The Endocrine Society and its Hormone Health Network, the map consists of a series of questions about your menopausal symptoms (hot flashes, vaginal dryness, interrupted sleep)...personal health (high blood pressure, diabetes, excess weight, unexpected spotting, etc.)...family medical history (cancer, blood clots)...and other factors. Based on your answers, it offers information on the various treatment options—lifestyle changes, botanical and vitamin supplements, topical and oral hormones—that may be appropriate for you. And it provides an individualized list of questions to ask your own physician...giving you an easy way to jump-start this important conversation.

Menopausal Fog

Miriam T. Weber, PhD, associate professor, department of neurology, University of Rochester Medical Center, Rochester, New York. Her study was published in *Menopause: The Journal of The North American Menopause Society*.

Many women look forward to reaching menopause and being freed from monthly menstrual hassles and worries about unintended pregnancy.

But they're not so happy if they find themselves experiencing menopausal "brain fog" —including poor concentration...difficulty recalling where they put things...and/or trouble remembering names and phone numbers.

And they're really not happy when their husbands and others get frustrated and blame them for forgetting things and just seeming to be "not all there."

Up to two-thirds of women say they experience brain fog while going through the midlife transition. And while some studies support this, there is not much objective proof of the phenomenon—so some people claim that the menopausal brain drain is all in women's heads, so to speak.

Researchers decided to find out whether menopausal brain fog is real...and, if so, to pinpoint exactly when a woman can expect it to start. *What they found was fascinating...*

HEAD TEST

To go hunting for brain fog, the researchers gathered 117 women, average age 49, and, based on each woman's stage of menopause, split them into four groups...

1. Late reproductive stage—characterized by subtle changes in menstrual flow and/or the length of menstrual cycles.

2. Early menopausal transition—a woman's cycles become persistently irregular, varying in length by a week or more.

3. Late menopausal transition—periods come two months or more apart.

4. Early postmenopause—the first 12 months after a woman's final period.

For the study, the women answered questionnaires about their general health, quality of life and symptoms (if any) of depression or anxiety. And they completed a battery of tests designed to measure their cognitive function—including their attention level...short-term or "working" memory...verbal fluency...dexterity...visual/spatial skill (for instance, identifying objects that had been cut into pieces and rearranged)...and verbal learning (such as recalling lists of words).

Results: Surprisingly, women in the third stage did just as well on the cognitive tests as those in the first and second stages, said lead researcher, Miriam T. Weber, PhD. However, women in the fourth stage (the first year after the final menstrual period) were a different story—for the most part, they did significantly worse on tests of attention, verbal memory, dexterity and verbal learning. For instance, Dr. Weber said, they took an average of five to six seconds longer to complete the dexterity task of putting pegs into pegboards...and they remembered an average of two fewer words in tests measuring recall of 15-word lists.

In other words, brain fog in postmenopausal women is real—and it seems to begin shortly after the last menstrual period.

HELLO, BRAIN FOG—NOW GO AWAY

The good news is that the cognitive dip seems to be temporary. Though Dr. Weber's research wasn't focused on measuring how long these effects persisted past menopause, a national women's health study done a few years ago suggested that cognitive skills rebound to premenopausal levels once a woman is postmenopausal. That study didn't specify exactly when the rebound takes place—but "postmenopausal" by definition means that a woman's final menstrual period occurred at least 12 months earlier.

Now, what can women do about all this? If you're heading into menopause, you're probably hoping to cope well with brain lapses while you wait for things to get back to normal. Weber offered these tips...

• **Safeguard your overall health.** Eating right, exercising, maintaining an appropriate weight and keeping blood pressure and cholesterol under control will help your brain work optimally.

• **Keep a calendar handy.** Write frequent notes to keep track of appointments and other commitments.

• **Resist the urge to multitask.** Focusing on one task at a time optimizes brain power—so turn off your cell phone and disable e-mail pop-up windows when you're in the middle of an important task.

• **Relax and be patient.** As Dr. Weber said, "Just knowing that this is a normal part of life might reduce anxiety, and that helps your brain function better."

Myth Buster: Thin Women Actually Have Fewer Hot Flashes

Because body fat can convert male hormones into estrogen, many people have long assumed that heavy women have an estrogen reserve that helps prevent menopausal hot flashes.

But: Recent research contradicts that notion. According to a study of 1,776 women ages 47 to 59, those who had a higher percentage of body fat were more likely to experience hot flashes and night sweats than those with less body fat.

Bottom line: If you are carrying extra pounds, try losing some weight. Not only will it improve your health, it just might help your hot flashes.

Rebecca C. Thurston, PhD, is an associate professor of psychiatry, epidemiology, psychology and clinical and translational science at the University of Pittsburgh, and leader of a study on weight and menopausal hot flashes.

Time to Switch Gynecologists?

Michelle P. Warren, MD, is founder and medical director of the Center for Menopause, Hormonal Disorders and Women's Health at New York–Presbyterian/Columbia University Medical Center in New York City and a nationally certified menopause practitioner.

You may have been using the same obstetrician/gynecologist for many years, perhaps even before your children were was born. Now that you're going through menopause, should you switch to a gynecologist who specializes in older women?

That is probably a good idea. Since your ob/gyn is in the business of delivering babies, she may not have time to stay on top of the scientific literature on menopause or the options for managing potential menopause-related problems. Menopause is a complex field, and our understanding of it is constantly growing. A thorough doctor/patient discussion of menopausal issues, such as the benefits and risks of hormone therapy, often takes much longer than a typical 15-minute office visit. Keep in mind, too, that physicians get scarcely any training about menopause in medical school—it is essentially just one lecture! If you go to a

doctor who isn't knowledgeable about this life transition, you will not get the same degree of attention to issues that can affect midlife and older women.

It is especially important to switch gynecologists if you do have bothersome menopausal symptoms—hot flashes, sleeplessness, moodiness, vaginal dryness and/or discomfort during sex—that are not getting addressed with your current doctor. To find a specialist, visit the website of the North American Menopause Society at *www.menopause.org*, click on "For Women" and then on "Find a Menopause Practitioner"

Acupuncture for Female Problems

Yi Hung Chan, DPM, LAc, lead acupuncturist, The Bendheim Integrative Medicine Center, Memorial Sloan Kettering Cancer Center, New York City. *YourDrChan.com*

Eleanor Walker, MD, Henry Ford Health System, Detroit, Michigan.

Acupuncture helps gynecological problems, including pain, infertility and menopause symptoms

Gynecological complaints like pelvic pain, infertility, menstrual cramps and the mood swings and hot flashes of menopause are often highly responsive to acupuncture—you may have heard this anecdotally from friends and, interestingly, also from doctors, both mainstream and integrative. Published research backs this up as well—recently, a 12-week study of breast cancer patients compared acupuncture treatment to use of an antidepressant, venlafaxine, for relief of severe hot flashes and other menopausal symptoms. Both treatments were effective, but with some important differences. The women in the acupuncture group reported no side effects, while the drug group suffered many unpleasant ones. The acupuncture group also reported improved energy, clarity of thinking, sexual desire and overall sense of well-being. Finally, improvement among the acupuncture patients lasted much longer—from three to four months after finishing treatment, compared with the Effexor group, in which symptoms resumed within two weeks after they stopped the drug.

WHY IT WORKS
FOR WOMEN'S ISSUES

We weren't surprised by any of this, given the many stories we've published about acupuncture, but it prompted us to look into the therapy's use for a wider range of gynecological issues. We spoke with acupuncturist Yi Chan, DPM, LAc, who is on staff at The Bendheim Integrative Medicine Center at Memorial Sloan-Kettering Cancer Center in New York and in private practice in West Orange, New Jersey. Dr. Chan says the basic philosophy of Chinese medicine is to maintain proper balance of energy flow (chi) in the body and that when the flow is disrupted, it creates disorders and discomfort. He likens this to the New York City subway where a breakdown of even a single train will cause widespread disruptions in the system. Acupuncture, he says, is a way to locate and correct the disruption of the chi.

Dr. Chan reports that acupuncture helps 80% of his patients—bringing "great improvement" to 60%. With acupuncture, most patients can tell by about the sixth treatment if it is helping their problem—if nothing has changed by then (as is true for about 20%), the challenge may be too great for acupuncture alone to resolve.

WHAT CAN
ACUPUNCTURE HELP?

• **Menstrual cycle problems (flow, regularity, pain).** Sometimes stress, diet or excessive exercise can disrupt normal functioning of the menstrual cycle, by sending energy to the wrong places, explains Dr. Chan. Acupuncture can help repair and "smooth out the bumpy ride," whether the flow is too heavy or too little, or the cycle is shortened, delayed or irregular. Typically, the practitioner treats the patient through several cycles, with about eight to 12 weeks of treatments.

• **Fertility issues.** Acupuncture can be helpful for women having trouble conceiving, and new research shows that it improves the success rate of in-vitro fertilization. Dr. Chan suggests not waiting many months to seek acupuncture to help fertility, urging women who don't get pregnant to use acupuncture sooner rather than later, as it can "free up" their energy flow. But such women should always first have a complete physical exam by a gynecologist to be sure that everything is anatomically functional.

• **Endometriosis and uterine fibroids.** These particular problems can be stubborn and complex. While acupuncture can help ease pain and excessive bleeding, women with endometriosis and/or fibroids often require conventional treatment as well, sometimes including surgery. In those cases, acupuncture can help soothe post-surgery discomfort, supporting healing and re-establishment of the cycle. Again, it is crucial to have a gynecological examination to determine the nature and extent of the problem—if symptoms are mild to moderate, Dr. Chan says acupuncture can help right away, but for severe symptoms, he says women should first see a medical doctor and then seek out an acupuncturist.

• **Hot flashes.** As mentioned above, acupuncture can ease the frequency and severity of hot flashes as well. Dr. Chan advises his patients to keep a notebook, writing down frequency and intensity of the flashes as they occur. With acupuncture, "the frequency may abate, but the intensity remains the same—or vice-versa," he says. "By observing this carefully you will know if acupuncture is working for you." Dr. Chan also has a list of "cooling" foods advised in Chinese medicine for such patients—watermelon, mung bean, mustard greens, bitter melon and grass jelly.

FIND AN ACUPUNCTURIST

To find an acupuncturist near you, go to the website of the National Certification Commission for Acupuncture and Oriental Medicine at *www.nccaom.org*, which lists board certified practitioners. Word of mouth is also good, says Dr. Chan. Insurance covers treatment in many cases, though not always. Perhaps this too will change as Western medicine begins to fully embrace the benefits of acupuncture.

Reducing Breast Cancer Risk After Menopause

JoAnn E. Manson, MD, MPH, DrPH, is a professor of medicine at Harvard Medical School and chief of the division of preventive medicine at Brigham and Women's Hospital, both in Boston. She is one of the lead investigators for two highly influential studies on women's health—the Nurses' Health Study and the Women's Health Initiative. Dr. Manson is author, with Shari S. Bassuk, ScD, of *Hot Flashes, Hormones & Your Health*.

Many postmenopausal women think their primary risk factor for breast cancer is genetics. Yet most breast cancers occur in women with no family history of the disease, and the major breast cancer genes (BRCA1 and BRCA2) account for only 5% to 10% of cases. *The primary risk factors...*

• **Age.** Average age at diagnosis is 61, and rates are highest after age 70.

• **Estrogen.** This hormone stimulates growth of breast tissues—including abnormal cells. Estrogen levels are highest during the childbearing years, so the earlier you started menstruating and the later you reached menopause, the higher your risk.

To help prevent breast cancer...

• **Guard against vitamin-D deficiency.** Vitamin D may fight formation of blood vessels that nourish tumors and inhibit division of cells that line the breast. Many experts now recommend that all adults get 1,000 international units (IU) daily.

Sources: Sunlight (from which skin synthesizes vitamin D)...cod liver oil, fatty fish (mackerel, tuna), fortified milk and cereals...and supplements of vitamin D3 (cholecalciferol).

• **Get adequate folate, a B vitamin involved in DNA synthesis and repair.** Eat three one-cup servings daily of folate-rich foods—leafy green vegetables, garbanzo beans, peas, citrus fruits.

• **Avoid unnecessary hormone therapy.** Consider taking estrogen (plus progestin to guard against uterine cancer, if you have not had a hysterectomy) only if hot flashes and night sweats significantly disrupt your sleep or quality of life. Use the lowest effective dose... try to limit use to less than four or five years.

• **Watch your weight.** Obesity after menopause may double breast cancer risk, perhaps because fat cells take over the ovaries' job of producing estrogen. Nearly one-quarter of postmenopausal breast cancers in the US are due to excess weight.

• **Exercise 30 minutes or more per day.** Exercise lowers blood levels of insulin and estrogen, both of which are risk factors for breast cancer.

• **Eat less saturated fat.** In a study of 48,835 postmenopausal women, those who were accustomed to a high-fat diet reduced their breast cancer risk by adopting a diet in which less than 25% of daily calories came from fat.

• **Limit alcohol intake.** Even moderate drinking raises breast cancer risk by increasing estrogen and decreasing folate absorption. Also, alcohol can be metabolized into acetaldehyde, a potential carcinogen, so have no more than one drink daily.

If you're at high risk: The drugs tamoxifen and raloxifene can reduce breast cancer risk—but increase the odds of blood clots, hot flashes, uterine cancer and perhaps stroke. Ask your doctor if these drugs are right for you.

13

Relationship Rx

The Secret to Relationship Happiness

A friend of mine has a husband who always leaves the kitchen cabinets open after he goes searching for, say, a box of cereal or crackers.

"I walk into the house and it feels like we've just been robbed," she told me. "But then I remember that it's just one of Bill's quirks."

If your partner has a similarly annoying habit, dealing with it can be frustrating. But there's an interesting tactic that can help you get past this sort of relationship frustration—you ready for it?

It involves something called Wabi Sabi.

Now, I'm not talking about that green, spicy stuff that you put on your sushi—I'm talking about the ancient Japanese principle of finding beauty in imperfections.

WHAT IS WABI SABI?

Picture the silhouette of a tree as the sun sets behind it, with its meandering, asymmetrical branches. It's beautiful. People who practice Wabi Sabi would say that the tree would be less beautiful if it were perfectly straight and symmetrical. They would also say that Cindy Crawford is beautiful because of the trademark mole above her lip, not in spite of it.

In reality, very few things in life (if any) are perfect, including marriages and long-term relationships. Practicing Wabi Sabi will help teach you how to manage your expectations when it comes to love—instead of expecting perfection from your partner and ending up feeling disappointed, you'll learn how to accept (and perhaps even adore) your partner's faults. As a result, you're likely to feel happier in your relationship.

Here are some of my favorite tips from the book that will help you reach that goal…

1. Learn to like what your partner loves. One common relationship frustration occurs

---

Arielle Ford, relationship expert based in La Jolla, California, and author of eight books, including *Wabi Sabi Love: The Ancient Art of Finding Perfect Love in Imperfect Relationships. WabiSabiLove.com*

126

when your partner is passionate about something (whether it's watching a sport, playing an instrument or going to a book club) and you have zero interest in it. The problem is that this passion can sometimes become all consuming and you may grow resentful if your partner spends more time pursuing that passion than he or she does with you!

For example, maybe it bothers you that your partner spends half the weekend on the sofa entranced by golf on TV. Instead of getting angry every time he starts getting settled in because he's not doing chores…or because you feel ignored…or because you think he's wasting his time, try sitting down and watching some golf with him. You may end up appreciating the precision of the players' shots, the energy of their competitive spirit or the serenity of the manicured courses. You don't need to love golf for the same reasons that he does, nor do you need to sit there for hours with him, but just being with him without steam coming from your ears—even for a few minutes—while he does something that he enjoys will help you understand why he loves it. The goal isn't to change your partner's behavior—it's to change your expectations and perspective, so you'll become more accepting of his habit.

2. Focus on the big picture. There is probably at least one thing that your partner does every day that makes you crazy—maybe she strikes up a conversation with every random stranger that she encounters, clicks her tongue as she reads the paper or leaves the toothpaste cap sitting on the bathroom counter next to the crumpled tube every single morning.

But in the grand scheme of things, when you think about your overall life together, are the annoying quirks really that terrible (or that important)? Try focusing on the major stuff instead of the minor stuff—meaning, be thankful for a moment that your partner is alive and well. There may come a day when your partner has passed away, and you may miss seeing the toothpaste cap on the counter or would do anything to hear that tongue clicking again.

3. Get some context. Here's a quick story: A guy named Jim punches a guy named Matt. Jim sounds like a jerk, right? But what if I told you that Matt had been having an affair with Jim's wife and had been stealing money from her to fund his gambling habit? This information might make you think about the punch—and Jim—in a different light, yes?

The point I'm trying to make is that context does matter. When you take the time to understand a person's frame of reference and see where he or she is coming from, you gain understanding and empathy. This strategy works wonders when it comes to relationships. Superstition, ethnic background, religion, family upbringing and a gazillion other things play a role in why your mate does certain things.

Say, for example, that your husband makes meat loaf every Monday for dinner. You're sick of looking at it and eating it and can't understand why he feels the need to make it so regularly.

Try this: Ask him why. Maybe it's because when he was growing up, that's what his mom did every Monday, and maintaining that ritual gives him comfort and reminds him of her. It's hard to stay annoyed at him when you know that, deep down, he's really doing it because he misses his mom.

Try to recall these three Wabi Sabi tips in your most important relationships. Hopefully you and your loved ones will experience more harmony and happiness together.

How to Be Best Friends with Your Grown Daughter

Karen L. Fingerman, PhD, is a psychologist and professor of human development and family sciences at the University of Texas at Austin's Population Research Center and author of *Mothers and Their Adult Daughters*. She serves on the editorial boards of the *Journal of Marriage and Family* and several other journals.

Did your grandmother ever tell you, "If you can't say something nice, don't say anything at all"? That seems to fly in the face of the advice we often hear today, which is to speak our minds openly. Yet when it comes to promoting positive relationships between mothers and adult daughters, Grandma's judicious lip-zipping is in fact a good policy, recent research suggests.

Researcher and psychologist Karen L. Fingerman, PhD, author of *Mothers and Their Adult Daughters*, explained that because it is a complex relationship, mother/daughter interaction can be fraught with tension. But navigating the turbulence is easier if you take your cue from another type of bond—the one you have with your girlfriends. Friendship provides an excellent model for a good relationship between mother and adult daughter, Dr. Fingerman said, because you learn to accept each other's flaws without confrontation. *What helps…*

• **Mind your own business.** After decades of motherhood, it can be hard to resist the urge to help your child become a "better person," Dr. Fingerman acknowledged—but your daughter may see your well-meant advice as critical and intrusive. Before you butt in, apply the friendship test. Would you tell a pal that her house was a mess or her hairstyle was frumpy? Not unless she asked…and even then, you would be tactful. Extend that same courtesy to your daughter.

• **Let go of disappointment.** Many moms wish that their grown kids would pay more attention to them. "But the fact is that mothers tend to rate their relationships with their adult daughters as being of much higher importance in their lives than the daughters do," Dr. Fingerman pointed out.

Test yourself: Compare your expectations for your daughter to what you would expect of a friend. Would you be upset if your friend didn't phone every week? Unlikely. "Most daughters are attentive to their mothers, but you should accept that your daughter has other demands on her time. She's not neglecting you when she doesn't call—she's just busy," Dr. Fingerman said.

Consider, too, whether resentment stems from a disappointment with yourself. For instance, if you scrimped to pay for your daughter's college and now feel let down because she's a stay-at-home mom instead of an executive, ask yourself whether your frustration is rooted in the regret that you never finished college or never pursued an office career. If

so, go get your degree or dream job now—and ask your daughter to provide encouragement as you pursue your goal. And remember to allow your daughter to make her own choices. After all, college provides many life lessons—not just career training.

Forgive yourself—as you would forgive a friend. Clinging to guilt over something that happened between you and your daughter years ago can limit closeness now, so remind yourself that you did what you thought was best at the time, Dr. Fingerman said. But don't pretend it never happened…even if it is harder to admit a mistake to your child than to a friend.

When Siblings Get Stuck in a Cold War

Judy Kuriansky, PhD, clinical psychologist and sex therapist on the adjunct faculty of Columbia University Teachers College in New York City. She is the author of several books, including *The Complete Idiot's Guide to a Healthy Relationship.* DrJudy.com

Betsy had barely spoken to her sister for several years. For a while, she was too angry about their last argument to mind the estrangement. Over time, though, as her ire mellowed, she started to miss her only sister. But she wasn't sure how to end the cold war, so she let month after month slip by without trying. Then she got the devastating news—her sister had passed away. Betsy had lost her chance to make peace…and now she's living with the heartache and regret.

Are you, too, experiencing a rift with a sibling? You don't have to make the same mistake Betsy made. If your sibling is truly toxic—for instance, if there is a history of abuse, criminal behavior or ongoing pathological selfishness that poisons every encounter—you may be better off keeping your distance. But otherwise, making the effort to rebuild sibling ties is likely to boost your own psychological health and improve the emotional well-being of the whole family. *Here's how to get started…*

● **First, figure out what's really behind the conflict.** On the surface, it may seem that the estrangement sprang from the most recent big fight. But chances are that its roots extend back to childhood, when you two saw yourselves as rivals for parental attention and affection.

Example: When your grown brother asked your parents for yet another "loan," you wrote him off as a leech and a loser—because you still resent the preferential treatment he always received as the "baby" of the family. Alternatively, you and your sibling may unconsciously repeat negative family patterns, mimicking the dysfunctional ways your parents treated each other. Whatever the true source of your sibling conflict, identifying it is the first step toward working through your feelings and finding healthier ways to interact.

● **Resolve to be the one who reaches out.** No matter who initiated the schism between you two, you can extend the olive branch. Yes, you may fear rejection—but don't let pride take precedence over peace. Remind yourself that life is too short to hold a grudge.

● **In reestablishing contact, appeal to your sibling's sense of nostalgia.** You might break the ice by sending your sibling a favorite old photo of the two of you together. Or mail a birthday card that expresses how much you miss the family connection. Or write a letter inviting your sibling to reconnect in light of an important life event that deserves to be shared, such as a parent's illness or the birth of a new grandchild. Don't give up too easily—if your first overture goes unacknowledged, wait a bit and then try again.

● **Acknowledge your own role.** Many people have trouble seeing the truth in this, but in the majority of cases, both parties contribute something to the conflict. Even if the bulk of the blame lies with your sibling, you probably played at least a small part. Admitting this to yourself lessens your resentment…acknowledging it to your sibling may make it easier for him or her to accept responsibility, too. Apologize sincerely—"I'm sorry that I teased you about your weight." Resist the urge to end with a "but" phrase (as in "but there was no reason for you to call me a nasty name, throw my favorite vase across the room and then refuse to speak to me for months"). Instead, end with a request for forgiveness—"Please pardon me for not giving you the respect you deserve."

● **Forge a new friendship.** Once contact has been renewed, strengthen ties by planning fun times together. Start small—for instance, with a siblings-only bike ride or an afternoon at a spa. While you're together, ask about your sibling's joys and concerns…truly listen to the responses and offer to help with a problem if possible. Remember, it's never too late to change the competitive, rivalrous relationship of childhood into one based on sharing and caring.

Mistakes Parents Make That Push Adult Children Away

Jeffrey Jensen Arnett, PhD, a research professor in the department of psychology at Clark University, Worcester, Massachusetts. He is coauthor, with Elizabeth Fishel, of *When Will My Grown-Up Kid Grow Up?* JeffreyArnett.com

Our children will always be our children, but once they turn 18 or leave home, they also are adults with lives increasingly separate from our own. It's a challenge for parents to step back while also staying connected to their grown-up kids.

Much of the angst between parents and adult children stems from the tug-of-war over whose life it is. There often is a disconnect between parents who still want to shape their grown-up kids' future course and the kids who are determined to live their lives their own way.

For loving parents, their grown children's trials and errors, including failed projects and teary breakups, can be anguishing. It can be wrenching to let go of the old parental omnipotence and not be able to fix everything. But when grown kids cope with these ups and downs, they develop into resilient, self-sufficient people with the confidence that comes from standing on their own feet.

Seven "don'ts" to keep in mind when dealing with grown children...

MONEY AND CAREER

It takes a long time these days for grown kids to achieve financial independence, and my research shows that money issues are the number-one topic of conflict between parents and kids 18 to 29 years old.

● **Don't use your financial support to control your adult kids.** If you're supplying money to your adult child, you certainly can set ground rules about how that money is used—but you should not threaten to withdraw your support if the adult child doesn't make life changes unrelated to finances.

Example: It's reasonable to tell your adult child that money you're providing cannot be spent on a vacation—but don't tell him that it can't be spent on a vacation unless he leaves the girlfriend you don't like.

● **Don't push your kids to take a job in a field that pays well but that they don't like.** Not only might they hold their unhappiness with the hated job against you, their lack of passion for the field could inhibit their career growth.

Also: Don't make snide comments about the job prospects of your college-age child's field of study or the earnings potential of his line of work. It is reasonable to discuss career and earnings outlooks with your kids before they choose a college major, field of graduate study or first job. But trying to control the big decision of what field your adult child will choose is sure to stir up resentment. Keep in mind that although college majors do vary in their future earnings, getting a college degree, in any area, is the most important goal for enhancing lifelong career prospects.

● **Don't insist that your kids find their own way after college rather than return home.** These days, many adult children live at home for a short time. Almost always, their return home is temporary because they prefer to live independently as soon as they can afford to do so.

Helpful: Agree on a division of household responsibilities. The adult child is now an adult member of the household and should do an adult share of the housework, laundry and cooking.

COMMUNICATION

Most adult children like talking to their parents and enjoy having a more adultlike relationship than they did in their teens. *But...*

● **Don't ask probing questions about your children's lives.** If they want to share something personal, they will. Adult children vary a lot in how much they want their parents to know about their lives and how much they want to confide in them.

Take special care not to raise subjects that your adult child has historically been disinclined to discuss. Resist the urge to ask follow-up questions on the rare occasions when your child does raise one of these subjects.

Example: Many adult children prefer not to discuss their love lives with their parents.

● **Don't overdo it.** Today's technology makes it cheap and easy to stay in contact with loved ones, and many adult children and their parents are in contact with one another nearly every day. However, for some grown kids, that's a bit too much togetherness at a time when they are striving to become self-sufficient. In general, it's best to follow your adult children's lead on communications. If they contact you weekly via text message, then contact them weekly via text message, too. Text messaging might not be your preferred communication method, but it's a great way to touch base with today's young adults without seeming pushy. You can always slip in a phone call now and then.

Helpful: Don't feel offended if kids go a few days without answering your text message or voice mail. It doesn't mean that they don't care. It could just mean that they are busy—or that they're not that eager to discuss that particular topic.

ROMANCE

An adult child's romantic relationships can be a minefield for parents...

● **Don't confide that you "never liked" an ex-boyfriend or ex-girlfriend or provide reasons why your adult child is better off**

without this former mate. Keep in mind that ex-boyfriends and ex-girlfriends sometimes re-enter the picture. That could create awkwardness if you've previously expressed a dislike.

•**Don't overlook your adult child's romantic partners at family get-togethers.** If your adult child has been seeing someone for a while, be sure to include the partner in family gatherings, then do your best to make him/her feel welcome and comfortable. The more comfortable your grown child's partner is with you, the more you are likely to see of your child.

BE CAREFUL WHEN IT COMES TO GIVING ADVICE

Many young adults spend their 20s acting in ways that seem irresponsible to their parents. They might change jobs or romantic partners frequently or rely on their parents for financial support or housing.

This is all perfectly normal and does not mean that the young adult is destined to act this way forever.

And while adult children might seem to be in desperate need of advice, there's a good chance that they will react poorly if their parents offer it. Such guidance makes them feel as if their parents still see them as children. This puts parents in a difficult position—they want to help their grown-up kids avoid missteps, but any wisdom they offer is likely to be poorly received.

Usually parents' best option is to bite their tongues and not offer their adult children advice when it hasn't been requested. Such advice might harm the relationship, and there is a good chance it won't be heeded anyway. *But speaking up could be wise if…*

•**You believe your adult child's safety is at risk.** It's worth putting the relationship at risk when safety is at stake.

Examples: Don't offer unsolicited advice if you think your adult child is staying out too late—but do if you suspect he's driving home drunk. Don't tell your daughter you don't like her new boyfriend—but do speak your mind if your daughter has a black eye and you suspect that the boyfriend is responsible.

•**The topic is money-related and you're providing financial support.** If your money is on the line, it's perfectly reasonable to voice concerns about the adult child's questionable financial decisions or even set ground rules for spending. But it will help the relationship if after voicing these concerns or setting these rules, you add something such as, "The final decision is yours, and I will continue to support you emotionally whatever you decide. I just can't continue to support you financially if you make this decision."

Example: You're paying your child's rent while he searches for a job, but you notice that he hasn't been looking for work lately. You obtain permission to provide advice. The odds of a negative reaction decline greatly if you ask the child if he would like your input before you offer it.

Warning: Respect the child's answer. If he says he prefers to work through the problem on his own, keep your advice to yourself. When you feel you must provide advice, also ask the adult child for his advice on a different topic about which he is knowledgeable. This can keep the relationship balanced.

How to Stay Close to Your Grown Kids

Scott Haltzman, MD, medical director, behavioral health department, St. Joseph's Medical Center, Providence. He is a psychiatrist in private practice in North Providence, Rhode Island, and author of *The Secrets of Happy Families: Eight Keys to Building a Lifetime of Connection and Contentment. DrScott.com*

In our mobile modern society, many adult children live hundreds or thousands of miles from their parents. Unfortunately, that geographical distance tends to be highly correlated with emotional distance from our kids and grandkids.

Even extended families whose members still live near one another face challenges, with ever-increasing demands on their time.

The good news: Parents can overcome these challenges and build strong relationships with their adult children no matter where they live. *Five ways to make that happen…*

SHOW RESPECT

Make your respect for your grown kids a recurring theme of the relationship. Adult children want one thing from their parents above all else—respect. The more you provide, the greater the odds that your children will want to remain close with you.

One way to show respect is to shower your grown kids with praise just as you did when they were young. Search for any excuse to offer a compliment. Make "I'm proud of you" and "You handled that very well" your mantras.

It also is important not to criticize your grown children when it seems as if they have failed. Criticism will only drive them away from you.

Helpful: If you catch yourself being critical, make at least five positive comments or actions before the end of your call or visit. Research has shown that a positive-to-negative interaction ratio of five-to-one or better can help maintain closeness in our relationships with our children (and our own spouses, too).

BUILD TRADITIONS

A family's traditions help to define it as well as preserve it. These traditions might include a distinctive way of celebrating a holiday or something as simple as gathering each year to watch an annual event on TV. Sure, your kids are busy with their own families and maybe there's been some bickering—but everyone still gathers at your house to watch the Super Bowl because it's a tradition.

It's never too late to create new family traditions. Whenever the extended family gets together and has a good time, single out something distinctive about the occasion—perhaps the place that the family gathered…the board game the family played…or the day of the year on which the gathering occurred. Suggest that the family try this again, perhaps the following year. If everyone has as much fun the second time, it could become a tradition.

Warning: Never make family traditions seem like requirements. If you hold it against your son that he spent Thanksgiving with his in-laws, the holiday could become a source of anxiety, driving your family apart, rather than a tradition that holds you together.

DON'T GIVE ADVICE

Resist the urge to give advice, even when it is requested. Receiving guidance from a parent can make adults feel like helpless children again. They tend to rebel against this unpleasant feeling by pulling away from the parent—even if they asked for advice.

If your adult child requests your advice, say, "I'm happy to help you sort through the pros and cons, but it's your decision to make, and I know you'll make the right choice."

One way to provide guidance to grown children is to ask them to teach you how they do something. Rather than criticize your adult children's decisions or methods, express an interest in these and ask if they could explain them to you. Listen attentively and without criticism, then casually mention that a different method was taught back when you were learning this task. Briefly describe your method and its advantages, then ask whether this strategy is still used. If your child doesn't wish to pursue the discussion any further, let it drop. This should dodge the psychological pitfalls of providing parental advice because the child gets to act as teacher first…and your guidance is presented as something that someone else taught you.

Example: When your son comes to you enthusiastically intending to buy junk bonds, you can ask about the company and its financial health, even look it up online with him. Then you can share how exciting it is to take a risk, as well as how you have learned not to invest any more than you can afford to lose.

Provide direct advice only if the adult child is about to make a massive and potentially irreversible misstep, such as driving an unsafe vehicle or buying an older home without a home inspection.

BEFRIEND YOUR CHILD'S SPOUSE

Search for ways to support and praise your sons- and daughters-in-law—even if you don't really care for them. It's your relationship with your children and grandchildren that will suffer the most if you don't get along with your kids' spouses. Your grown kids might decide it's easier to cut you out of their lives than to deal with the problems created when you and the spouse are together. And your child's spouse is likely to come up with excuses for the child's family not to visit you or invite you over.

Warning: The fact that your child criticizes his/her spouse to you does not mean that you are free to criticize that spouse, too. What you take as serious criticisms might just be your child venting normal marital frustrations. He actually might love and respect this partner very deeply. If so, your criticisms might damage your relationship with your child.

DON'T INTRUDE

Select noninvasive communication methods. Frequent phone calls or drop-in visits from parents can seem overbearing to adult children. *Better options…*

•**E-mail and social-networking websites.** Modern technology lets families keep in touch without interfering with one another's schedules. You can write as much as you like in an e-mail message or on a Facebook page—and your kids can read it whenever they like.

•**Care packages.** Young kids away at summer camp aren't the only ones who appreciate care packages. A batch of cookies that arrives unexpectedly in the mail can be a great way to remind your adult child of your love. My mother sent me clothes that she found on sale for a full decade after I married. My wife and I both appreciated it.

Warning: Do not follow up your packages with calls. These calls could make it seem like you are fishing for a thank-you or an invitation to visit. Gifts are most effective as relationship builders when there are no strings attached.

Also, be sure that gifts won't be misconstrued as subtle hints that your children or their spouses don't measure up. Books about dieting or a free session with a marriage counselor will be seen by your kids as signs of your disapproval, even though in your eyes, you're just trying to help.

When Grown Kids Move Back Home— Living (Happily) Together

John L. Graham, PhD, professor of marketing and international business, University of California, Irvine. He is coauthor, with Sharon Graham Niederhaus, of *Together Again: A Creative Guide to Successful Multigenerational Living.*

In these economic times, more grown children are moving back home. The arrangement can work well for you and your child if you discuss expectations and ground rules upfront.

•**Set a deadline.** If you do not want your child to stay indefinitely, say so. You may want to extend the offer only until the child meets a goal.

Examples: Earning a degree…saving for a down payment on a home…recovering from an illness…or finding a job.

•**Decide if your adult child will pay rent and what expenses he/she will cover.** Many parents don't charge rent as long as the child is pursuing mature goals, such as saving money or getting an education. However, if your money is tight and your child is working, it's not unreasonable to expect him to contribute a fixed sum monthly. Adult children usually pay for any extras they need, such as a separate phone/computer line.

•**Limit babysitting.** Be explicit about your limits in caring for grandchildren who come to live or visit. You may want to limit it to, say, two mornings or one night a week. If you want the overall experience to be a good one, you will need to respect your child's choices in child-rearing and avoid critical remarks.

•**Knock before entering.** Agree on the appropriate rules for entry into one another's private spaces. Do not open your adult child's mail, read his e-mail or answer his cell phone without his okay. He should extend the same courtesy to you.

•**Talk about whether it's acceptable to discuss each other's health, finances and**

relationships with other people, and with whom. Also, make specific agreements about visitors, boyfriends/girlfriends and parties.

• **Split the chores.** Adult children typically clean their own living spaces, do their own laundry and take care of their own pets.

Shared chores that tend to cause stress: Moving heavy trash cans…sorting and picking up the mail from shared mailboxes…and moving the car when parking is an issue. Perhaps alternate these tasks or assign them to the person who doesn't mind doing them.

• **Use a headset.** Families often find it desirable to use headsets for listening to radio, television and music so that they don't need to adjust to one another's taste and preferred volume.

• **Meet regularly.** After your child moves in, meet regularly—monthly is usually about right—with the specific purpose of discussing how the current rules are working. I know a mother, father and grown son who have their meeting on a weekend walk. For larger families, meetings may need to be more businesslike. Keep the meeting short, agreeing in advance on the ending time. The organizer begins by asking everyone what is working well before turning to problems. Encourage compromise and creative thinking on all sides.

How to Get Anyone to Like You in Two Minutes or Less

Leil Lowndes, a communications consultant and corporate trainer based in New York City, whose clients have included Temple University, Kodak and the US Peace Corps. She is author of *How to Instantly Connect with Anyone. Lowndes.com*

If you want to make new friends or land new clients or a new job, you need to make a great first impression—fast. People form permanent opinions of those they meet within just a few minutes of setting eyes upon them.

A study published in *Journal of Experimental Psychology: General* reported that the first impression someone has of a new acquaintance is likely to always dominate the way he/she views this acquaintance. Any later evidence that this first impression might have been erroneous tends to be dismissed as nothing more than an exception to the rule.

The trouble is, making a good first impression can be tricky. Our words, actions, facial expressions and body language all send subtle messages, often without our even realizing that we are doing it.

Below are 11 tricks for making a great first impression. Pick just one or two to try at a time, and add more when those become second nature.

YOUR BODY AND FACE

Facial expression and body position can make you seem more likable to those you meet…

1. Use a slow-flooding smile. Obviously it's a good idea to smile when you meet someone, but instantly switching on a 100-watt smile can make you seem phony. Instead, let your smile build slowly when you make eye contact. This sends the message that there is something about this person in particular that you like.

2. Have "sticky" eyes. People are inclined to like and trust those who make strong eye contact. If you are not a natural at maintaining eye contact, make it a habit to note specific characteristics about new acquaintances' eyes—what color are they…what shape…how far apart…how long are their lashes…how often do they blink…how often do they look away while talking to you? Answering these questions will force you to make strong eye contact with the other person.

Do break eye contact occasionally—staring too intently can make people uncomfortable—but don't do it abruptly. Break eye contact slowly, as if your gaze were stuck on this person and you find it difficult to pull it away.

3. Select an open, welcoming body position. Arrange yourself so that your torso is mostly but not completely facing the person whom you just met. During the first minute of conversation, very slowly and slightly rotate your body to completely face this person.

Exception: A man meeting a woman for the first time should stop a few degrees short of angling his upper body directly toward hers. That seems overly aggressive to some women.

If you are holding a drink or plate of hors d'oeuvres, either find a spot to set it down or hold it down by your side. If you hold it up in front of your chest, your arm will block off your body, making you seem less open. If you are self-conscious about what to do with your hands, use gestures when you talk or even put your hands in your pockets—just don't cross your arms across your chest, which makes you seem closed off.

4. Stand with one foot a few inches forward of the other. Put most of your weight on the forward foot. This stance suggests that you're an energetic person and are interested in the person with whom you are speaking.

YOUR ACTIONS

Even seemingly inconsequential actions can affect how you are viewed during an initial meeting…

5. Find your conversation partner's personal-space comfort zone. Stand too close to a new acquaintance, and you will make him feel uncomfortable. Stand too far away, and the odds increase that he will not feel a connection with you. What's the proper distance? For the average American, it's around 24 inches. Trouble is, that's just an average—everyone is a little different.

The best strategy is to start a conversation with a new acquaintance by placing yourself 26 to 28 inches away. Move toward this person imperceptibly slowly until you see discomfort in his eyes. Then ease back very slightly until that discomfort disappears.

6. When you shake hands, very gently touch your forefinger to the other person's wrist. Aim for the spot on the underside of the wrist where you would take a pulse. This is a very sensitive spot, and gently touching it tends to foster a feeling of warmth and closeness, even though your light contact might not be consciously noticed by the other person. Attempting this wrist touch also forces a deep handshake, which encourages a sense of closeness, too.

7. Treat business cards with respect. A business card symbolizes someone's professional accomplishments. Showing respect for the card shows respect for the person. When you are handed a card, imagine that it is a delicate and precious gift. Hold it gently in your hands. Pause to read it, then carefully place it into your briefcase or purse or, at the very least, your wallet. Never just jam a card into a pocket.

YOUR WORDS

A few tips for an initial conversation…

8. Begin with a conversation starter question or two. Questions that make great ice-breakers include, "What do you do?" followed by "How did you decide that you wanted to do that?"…Or (to couples) "How did you two meet?"

9. Slowly nod while people speak. This sends a message of acceptance and encouragement, which makes people feel more in sync with us.

Important: Be aware that men and women can have different interpretations of nodding. Do not nod if a man is saying something with which you completely disagree. Your nodding might be interpreted as agreement. Women, however, tend to interpret nodding as meaning, "I understand," not "I agree."

10. Listen for words that suggest people's interests. The words that people use and the topics that they reference, even in passing, often provide hints at their true areas of interest. If you can spot these words and topics, you can redirect dull, forgettable small-talk conversations toward things that people actually want to talk about.

Examples: If the small talk is about the weather and someone says, "At least the rain is good for my plants," seize on the word plants and ask, "Do you have a garden?" If someone says, "It's been too hot to walk my dogs," seize on the word dogs and ask "What kind of dogs do you have?"

11. Use the same terms as your conversation partner. This is particularly important when discussing topics that tend to matter to a lot of people, such as their families or careers.

Examples: If a parent refers to her "child," you should ask about her "child" as well, not her "little one" or "baby." If someone refers to his "profession," you should refer to it as his "profession," not his "job" or "career."

People tend to use the terms that their family members or closest friends use. If you use the same terms, it increases the odds that this person will feel comfortable with you.

Right Way to Give Advice

Judy Kuriansky, PhD, clinical psychologist and sex therapist on the adjunct faculty of Columbia University Teachers College in New York City. She is author of several books, including *The Complete Idiot's Guide to a Healthy Relationship*. DrJudy.com

Unless it is carefully worded, advice can offend. *What's hurtful, what's helpful…*

Hurtful: "You should." If you tell your friend to get out of that marriage, he may get angry if this isn't what he wants to hear…or feel pressured if he's not ready to follow through.

Helpful: Ask questions that encourage clarification of facts and feelings, such as, "If you left, where would you go?" and "How would the kids react?" This helps elicit your own choice—at which point your suggestions for implementing that decision will be appreciated.

Hurtful: "I had that problem." If you interrupt a friend's story ("I felt a lump in my breast once, too…"), she feels alone because you're not focusing on her.

Helpful: Ask for details and offer practical assistance—"When is your biopsy? May I drive you?" Only after discussing her situation completely should you share your experience and counsel.

Hurtful: "You'll get over it." To move past a problem, a person must face up to it, not avoid it. If a friend loses his job, and your automatic response is, "Stop fretting…you will find something better," ask yourself why. Are you too worried about your own job security to think about another's situation?

Helpful: Allow your friend to fully voice the hurt—afterward you'll both feel more ready to explore opportunities that lie ahead.

Expanding Your Circle of Friends

Judy Kuriansky, PhD, clinical psychologist and sex therapist on the adjunct faculty of Columbia University Teachers College in New York City. She is author of several books, including *The Complete Idiot's Guide to a Healthy Relationship*. DrJudy.com

Two tickets to your favorite opera just fell into your lap, but no one you know shares your passion for arias. Or you need to get something upsetting off your chest but fear that none of your usual confidantes would really understand. Or maybe you're just a bit bored being at home by yourself and wish you had more pals to hang out with.

Whatever your reason for feeling alone, the solution is to find some more new friends. *Here's how to get started…*

• **Go to places where you'll see the same people repeatedly.** Familiarity fosters friendship. Clubs and classes provide the opportunity for repeat encounters that promote increasing comfort with and connection to fellow members. As a bonus, they also guarantee a shared interest upon which to build a bond. So: Register for that fascinating history course at the local community college…sign up for that spin class you've been meaning to try…or join your town's gardening club.

• **Pursue activities that invite interaction.** You may love going to the movies or the theater, but a dark auditorium is not a great venue for getting a conversation going.

Better: Go to lectures about movies, where people will be exchanging ideas…or join a community theater or improv group, where participants naturally get to know each other on personal levels. Or if sports are your passion, don't just stay home alone to watch games on

TV. Instead, go to a local restaurant where the games are broadcast or, better yet, become a booster for a local team. The high-energy environment at the restaurant or playing field helps dissipate shyness and encourages strangers to interact enthusiastically with fellow fans. You don't even have to spend big bucks to see professional athletes—your local school teams would welcome your support.

• **Take a fresh look at current acquaintances.** Sure, it's great to meet new people, but don't be too quick to dismiss those you already know in passing. Your initial indifference (for instance, to the foreign-born coworker who never laughs at your jokes) or even aversion (to the neighbor who looks like the vixen who stole your high school boyfriend) might be un-warranted. Challenge yourself to see beyond superficial characteristics to recognize that a person with a different outlook or background can provide a refreshing change of pace as a new pal.

• **Make the first move.** Once you've found another woman with whom you'd like to be closer, show that you're interested and can be counted on. Pass along a book she had mentioned wanting to read or a CD you think she'd enjoy…invite her to go for a bike ride or to come by your house to sample a new recipe you discovered…offer to walk her dog or run an errand for her when she's feeling overwhelmed or under the weather. Remember, the easiest way to make a good friend is to be a good friend.

14

Sex and Intimacy

Great Sex, Naturally—Women: Revive Your Sex Drive

Diminished libido—little or no sexual desire—is the most common sexual complaint among women. But repeated attempts by the pharmaceutical industry to solve the problem with one or another form of "female Viagra" have failed.

My viewpoint: Reviving a mature woman's sex drive requires addressing multiple factors. *These include…*

Balancing hormones—which play a key role in both physical and mental aspects of arousal—particularly during the hormonal changes of perimenopause and menopause.

Treating the pelvic problems of aging, such as vaginal atrophy and dryness, which can cause painful sex.

Here are natural ways to boost libido that consistently work for the mature women in my medical practice. Choose one or two based on your particular needs. If you still have problems, consult a licensed naturopathic physician.

HORMONE HELP

Several herbs and herbal combinations can help balance a mature woman's hormones. *Two of my favorites…*

•**Maca.** This powerful Peruvian herb is a good choice for women going through perimenopause or menopause because it is rich in plant sterols that balance and strengthen the entire hormonal system. The herb not only increases sex drive but also improves perimenopausal and menopausal symptoms such as hot flashes, night sweats and insomnia. Additionally, it supports the adrenal glands, reducing levels of energy-depleting stress hormones.

Laurie Steelsmith, ND, LAc, a licensed naturopathic physician and acupuncturist with a 20-year private practice in Honolulu. Dr. Steelsmith is coauthor of *Great Sex, Naturally: Every Woman's Guide to Enhancing Her Sexuality Through the Secrets of Natural Medicine.* DrLaurieSteelsmith.com

Typical dose: 1,000 milligrams (mg), twice daily.

● **Two Immortals.** This herbal formula from Traditional Chinese Medicine builds two types of chi, or life-energy—yin (feminine) chi and yang (masculine) chi—thereby boosting a woman's libido, which requires both nurturing (yin) and stimulation (yang).

It also helps to balance hormones and control some symptoms of perimenopause (irregular menstrual bleeding and cramping) and menopause (hot flashes).

Many of my patients take it for six months to a year to rebuild their vitality.

Typical dose: Many companies manufacture the supplement, and dosages vary—follow the dosage recommendation on the label.

SUPER-SEX SUPPLEMENTS

Two nutritional supplements are particularly effective at stimulating sexuality…

● **L-arginine.** This amino acid works by boosting nitric oxide, a compound that promotes blood flow—including blood flow to your genitals.

A study in *Journal of Sex & Marital Therapy* showed that more than 70% of women who took a supplement containing L-arginine (ArginMax for Women) experienced increased sexual desire, more frequent sex and orgasm, enhanced clitoral stimulation, decreased vaginal dryness and improved overall sexual satisfaction.

Typical dose: 3,000 mg daily.

Caution: Talk to your doctor before you take L-arginine, especially if you have low blood pressure, herpes, gastric ulcer, liver disease or kidney disease.

● **PEA (phenylethylamine).** Called the "love supplement," PEA boosts the neurotransmitter dopamine, enhancing feelings of well-being, joy and pleasure.

Typical dose: 60 mg once a day. (Higher doses can cause overstimulation, insomnia or anxiety.)

Caution: Don't take PEA if you're nursing, pregnant or take an MAOI antidepressant medication such as *selegiline* (Eldepryl).

You also can boost PEA by exercising regularly, eating dark chocolate and taking a blue-green algae called spirulina.

APHRODISIACS

Two aphrodisiacs are particularly effective for mature women because—by relaxing your body and improving your mood—they slowly and gently boost your libido.

● **Cordyceps.** This mushroom is considered a potent sexual tonic in Traditional Chinese Medicine. It enhances both yin and yang chi, making it an ideal aphrodisiac for women.

Typical dose: 500 mg, twice daily.

What works best: Pills made by a hot-water extraction process that pulls out the herb's most active constituents, such as the cordyceps supplement from JHS Natural Products.

● **Ginkgo biloba.** Often recommended for memory loss because it improves blood supply to the brain, ginkgo also promotes blood flow to the vulva and vagina. Studies show that it may help restore libido in women taking antidepressants, which can destroy sex drive.

Typical dose: 40 mg, three times a day. The label should read, "Standardized extract of 24% ginkgo flavonglycosides (or flavone glycosides)."

STATIN WARNING

Cholesterol-lowering statin drugs—taken by millions of older women—can lower libido, probably by damaging mitochondria, energy-generating structures inside cells. If you take a statin and notice a decrease in libido, talk to your doctor about your options.

VAGINAL WEIGHT-TRAINING

The pubococcygeal (PC) muscle—a bowl-shaped "hammock" of pelvic muscle that contracts rhythmically when you have an orgasm and also supports your genital organs and bladder—is crucial to sexual pleasure.

New approach: Using a vaginal weight (a small, round weight inside an oval tube that is inserted into the vagina like a tampon) is the best way to strengthen the PC muscle, enhancing erotic sensation and sexual response.

What to do: To start, insert the tube for one to five minutes, twice daily, squeezing your PC muscle repeatedly to hold the tube in place. You can do this standing or lying down. Gradually work up to 20 minutes, twice daily, using progressively heavier weights. Do this for three months. You can order a set of vaginal weights at *www.Vagacare.com*.

Cost: About $35.

Other benefits: Regular use of vaginal weights can help prevent and treat urinary incontinence and prevent prolapse of the bladder or uterus.

VAGINAL DRYNESS AND PAINFUL INTERCOURSE

Enjoyable sex requires vaginal tissue that is healthy and well-hydrated. But the midlife drop in estrogen levels causes a decrease of blood flow to the vagina, which can lead to vaginal atrophy and dryness. A simple remedy...

• **Vitamin E.** The unique lubricating properties of vitamin E make it especially effective.

What to do: Pierce a soft 400 IU vitamin E gel capsule with a pin, squeeze the oil onto your finger, and apply it to the outside of the vagina and inside about an inch. Or use a vitamin E vaginal suppository. (I recommend the product from Earth's Botanical Harvest, available online.) Apply the gel or insert the suppository nightly at bedtime for at least two weeks. Taper use to three times a week.

How to Be a Better Lover

Lou Paget, a sex educator certified by the American Association of Sexuality Educators, Counselors and Therapists. Based in Los Angeles, she is host of the radio program *Sex Talk with Lou* and a regular speaker at national and international professional conferences. She is author of five books, including *The Great Lover Playbook*. Her website is *LouPaget.com*.

The secret to being a great lover is not necessarily a matter of knowing exotic techniques in the bedroom. It is more about developing an attitude of openness and curiosity—and making a commitment to keeping passion alive. *Here's how anyone can be a better lover...*

SHOW APPRECIATION

When we show appreciation, it creates good feelings, which draws us closer to our partner. Often we notice something about our partner that pleases us, but we don't think to say anything. Instead, speak up.

Example: "I really admire the way you stood up to your boss. That took guts."

Even better, tell others how proud you are of your partner, in your partner's presence. Champion your lover.

Example: "Have you heard about the fund-raising drive she organized? She did an amazing job." Bragging about other people isn't offensive if it is obvious that you take genuine pleasure in their achievements and aren't just trying to impress others.

Both men and women enjoy being told they are attractive. When she wears that dress that shows off her body, tell her how great she looks. When he steps out of the shower, tell him how sexy he is.

PAY ATTENTION

Pure, nondistracted attention is affirming and seductive. When your partner tells you about his/her thoughts, feelings, desires or just the things that happened that day, stop what you're doing and really listen. Don't keep tapping on your computer keyboard or have one eye on the television.

Another way to pay attention is to show that you are thinking of your partner. Make a cup of coffee for her while she is in the shower, and clear the snow off her car. Call him during the day to tell him you love him and let him know about an article you read in the paper that you think he would find useful. Draw her a bath with lavender bath salts when she comes home from work.

BE ADVENTUROUS

Shake up your routine so that you see each other with new eyes. If you have fallen into the habit of cuddling on the couch and watching DVDs on the weekend, take a day trip instead or invite friends over for dinner. Exchange chores for a week.

Bring a sense of adventure to everyday events. Point out to each other the birds that are visiting the backyard bird feeder or the trees that are budding in your neighborhood. The ongoing accumulation of shared experiences, small and large, builds your shared personal history and increases intimacy.

PLAN CLOSENESS

Although planning may seem to work against adventure and spontaneity, the opposite is true. If you think about the times when so-called spontaneous sex happened, it was most likely possible because of planning—whether for a dinner date or a luxurious vacation. This planning doesn't necessarily mean planning sex—it means taking the time to create an environment conducive to intimacy.

TOUCH

Touching is the most powerful way to connect. It releases the "love hormone" oxytocin. The more you touch each other, the more you will desire each other. Give each other massages...cuddle first thing in the morning... pause for a full-body embrace as one of you is going out the door...take his arm or place your hand on the small of her back as you are walking...hold hands before going to sleep.

Be aware that men need to be touched two to three times more frequently than women to maintain the same level of oxytocin, according to a study by Swedish researchers.

AVOID PSYCHIC SEX

Many people believe that they should be able to intuit what will make a partner happy in bed. But it is dangerous to assume that you can figure out what your partner wants without asking. You may wind up focusing on activities that you enjoy but that your partner does not and vice versa.

It is helpful to have this conversation in broad daylight so that you can see your partner's face and subtle reactions. If you are self-conscious about raising the topic, try doing so when you are lying down and snuggling, with low lighting—but not in the middle of sex. You can say, "You know, I was reading an article and realized that there are some things I don't know about what you enjoy in bed. I would love to know more, because I want to create that kind of pleasure for you. And I'd

love to tell you about some things that sound exciting to me."

If your partner is shy and doesn't offer ideas, you could suggest a particular activity and say, "I thought this might be fun to try. Do you think you would like it, or is there a variation you might like more?"

If your lover has been touching you in a way that you don't enjoy anymore, speak in terms of your nerves and sensations. This keeps the information from feeling like a personal criticism.

Example: "You know, it's almost like this has a different sensation for me—I might like it a little lighter or more on this side."

KISS CREATIVELY

Kissing is one of the least threatening, and most exciting, ways to vary your intimacy. But couples fall into a pattern where they essentially stop kissing or kiss in the same way, in the same places, time after time. Instead, experiment with playful Eskimo kisses (nose to nose)...kiss your partner's lips in a new way... explore your partner's body with your mouth.

One way to let your lover know what style of kissing you like is to begin kissing him/her the way you enjoy being kissed. Pause in mid-kiss and say, "Mmm, I love the way this feels." Then say, "Hey, would you show me what it feels like to be kissed by me just now?" Reinforce by saying, "Oh, do more of that."

STIMULATE YOUR SENSES

Engage all your senses—smell, hearing, touch, taste and sight. Light scented candles... play pulsating music or the song that was playing when you met...put fresh sheets on the bed...feed each other foods that you find aphrodisiacal (anything from oysters to chocolate-covered strawberries)...put a different-colored bulb in the bedside lamp.

Herbal Love Potions with Proof to Back Them Up

Laurie Steelsmith, ND, LAc, a licensed naturopathic physician and acupuncturist with a 20-year private practice in Honolulu. Dr. Steelsmith is coauthor of *Great Sex, Naturally: Every Woman's Guide to Enhancing Her Sexuality Through the Secrets of Natural Medicine. DrLaurieSteelsmith.com*

Countless "natural love potions" purportedly provide a boost in the bedroom, online ads proclaim. But many of them are bunk...because if you dig deeper, you'll find that only a few herbal sex enhancers are backed up with scientific evidence of effectiveness.

We discussed this with naturopathic physician Laurie Steelsmith, ND, LAc, coauthor of *Great Sex, Naturally: Every Woman's Guide to Enhancing Her Sexuality Through the Secrets of Natural Medicine.* Fortunately, she said, the few proven herbal remedies address three of the most common sex complaints among midlife and senior adults—low libido, erectile problems and antidepressant-induced sexual dysfunction.

The following herbal products are sold over the counter in health-food stores and online. However, before you try them, Dr. Steelsmith recommended seeing a licensed naturopathic physician to discuss your health history (because treating an underlying medical disorder could solve the sex problem)...to ensure that the herbs are safe and appropriate for you (because they can cause side effects and/or interact with certain medications)...and to get specific dosage instructions. For a referral, visit the website of the American Association of Naturopathic Physicians at *www.Naturopathic. org. Here's how herbs can help with...*

• **Low libido.** "Not tonight, dear, I have a headache," is a classic punch line—but loss of libido is no joke, especially considering how common it is. In a recent AARP survey of adults ages 45 and older, only a scant 6% of female respondents said that they had a higher-than-average level of sexual desire, while a whopping 40% of women said that they had a lower-than-average libido.

Studies involving postmenopausal women show that Panax ginseng (also called Korean or Asian ginseng) can improve arousal, possibly due to its relaxing effects on clitoral and vaginal muscles. "Ginseng modulates the nervous system, boosting sexual energy if you're lethargic and helping you relax when stress dampens your libido," Dr. Steelsmith said. An alternative she recommended is the brand-name product ArginMax for Women (*www.Ar ginMax.com*), which contains ginseng plus the herb ginkgo biloba and the amino acid L-arginine (both of which promote circulation) and vitamins and minerals (for general wellness). Dr. Steelsmith generally advises her patients to try ginseng or ArginMax for three months to see whether it helps restore libido...if so, it can be used as long as desired.

Caution: Side effects may include diarrhea, restlessness, vertigo, breast pain and/or menstrual changes. Avoid ginseng if you have hot flashes, insomnia, dry mouth, dry skin, high blood pressure, a heart rhythm disorder or a bleeding disorder—it could exacerbate symptoms.

• **Erectile dysfunction (ED).** OK, so this is a guy's problem—but that makes it a problem for us women, too. In the AARP survey, erectile problems were reported by 13% of men in their 40s...18% in their 50s...38% in their 60s...and 56% in their 70s or beyond.

Encourage your partner to talk to his doctor about yohimbine, the active ingredient in the extract of the bark of the yohimbe tree. Studies show that it helps ED by increasing blood flow to the penis and stimulating the central nervous system and genital nerves. Generally it is taken daily (not just prior to sex the way an ED drug would be used), continuing indefinitely.

Caution: Do not exceed the dosage recommend by a doctor or listed on the product label. Yohimbine may cause restlessness, irritability or other side effects. Yohimbe should not be used by men who take MAO inhibitors or blood thinners or who have cardiovascular disease, blood pressure problems or seizure disorders, Dr. Steelsmith said.

• **Antidepressant-induced sexual dysfunction.** Among AARP survey respondents, 16% of women and 10% of men were taking antidepressant medication. For both women and men, these drugs are notorious for causing sexual side effects—decreased genital sensation, low libido, erectile problems and/or difficulty reaching orgasm.

The herb gingko can help counter such side effects. It has demonstrated positive effects on all four phases of the sexual response cycle—desire…arousal (lubrication in women and erection in men)…orgasm…and resolution (afterglow). For patients on antidepressants, Dr. Steelsmith usually advises daily use of a gingko extract labeled "standardized to 24% of ginkgo flavone glycosides," continuing for as long as a patient is on antidepressant medication. Ginkgo generally is well-tolerated, though occasionally it may cause stomach upset, headache or restlessness.

Caution: Because it may increase bleeding risk, gingko should not be used by patients who take a blood thinner, are anticipating surgery or are pregnant.

Sex After a Long Dry Spell

Barbara Bartlik, MD, is a sex therapist and assistant clinical professor of psychiatry at Weill Cornell Medical College in New York City. She is the author of numerous scientific publications and medical advisor for the book *Extraordinary Togetherness: A Woman's Guide to Love, Sex and Intimacy.*

I*'ve been without a partner for a long time, but now I'm starting a new relationship. Since I haven't been intimate for years, is sex going to hurt?*

Intercourse is likely to be uncomfortable at first because the vagina can atrophy from lack of activity. Also, if you are postmenopausal, vaginal tissues can become thin and dry due to the natural decline in estrogen and testosterone levels, exacerbating the discomfort of penetration. Fortunately, there is a lot you can do now to prepare yourself so that intercourse will be enjoyable. *Try any or all of the following…*

•**Start using a nonhormonal over-the-counter vaginal moisturizer,** which is a topical suppository, cream or gel with long-lasting effects. Routinely applied two or three times per week, it helps rejuvenate the vaginal tissues, making them more moist and resilient.

Good brand: Replens.

•**Once daily, use a pin to pierce a vitamin E gel-cap supplement (500 IU),** squeeze the oil onto your fingertips, then rub it onto the labia and around the vaginal opening. This plumps up and strengthens the cells.

•**Ask your gynecologist whether a prescription topical estrogen cream or suppository is appropriate for you.** Topical estrogen can improve the integrity of the vaginal lining, reducing the chances of tearing and lessening any discomfort you might experience during sex—and because very little gets into the bloodstream, it does not carry the same level of risk for systemic side effects as oral estrogen does. (Topical estrogen generally is not recommended for women at high risk for breast or ovarian cancer, but there are exceptions.) Also ask about specially compounded testosterone cream to be applied to the vulva. Though not FDA-approved for this purpose, doctors have been prescribing this to women for many years.

•**Keep a water-based or silicone-based personal lubricant on hand so you'll have it when you need it.** Used during foreplay and intercourse, it helps minimize pain and heighten pleasure. Some lubricants contain ingredients that can irritate delicate tissues, particularly in menopausal women, so look for a product that is organic, hypoallergenic and/or paraben-free.

Excellent brands include Hathor Aphrodisia, Pink and Sliquid.

•**Do Kegel exercises, aiming for 20 minutes or 200 repetitions per day.** Repeatedly squeezing and then releasing the muscles you use to start and stop the flow of urine can increase the flow of blood, oxygen and nutrients to the pelvic floor, strengthening not only the muscles but also the tissues in that area.

Bonus: Kegels help prevent incontinence and may intensify orgasms.

- **Masturbate on your own, with a vibrator if desired,** to rediscover what makes you feel aroused. Sometimes getting back in the game takes practice.

- **Consider talking to your gynecologist about a vaginal dilator,** which is a set of smooth cylindrical probes in varying sizes. You use the dilator at home to gradually stretch the vagina—so that by the time you want to have intercourse, you are physically ready.

Pleasure-Enhancing Feminine Parts You Never Knew You Had

Laurie Steelsmith, ND, LAc, a licensed naturopathic physician and acupuncturist with a 20-year private practice in Honolulu. Dr. Steelsmith is coauthor of *Great Sex, Naturally: Every Woman's Guide to Enhancing Her Sexuality Through the Secrets of Natural Medicine. DrLaurieSteelsmith.com*

Countless women have pored over the book *Our Bodies, Ourselves*, starting when it first came out in the 1970s and continuing right up through the most recent edition published in 2011. When my generation first read it decades ago, getting to know the intricacies and intimacies of our sexual selves seemed like a radical idea. These days, I'd venture to say, we women tend to be well-acquainted with our sex organs.

Even so, you may be surprised by how much more there is to learn, particularly about the hidden parts—and how much pleasure that new knowledge can bring.

Bonus: Better sex often leads to a better relationship.

For details I consulted the perfect expert source, Laurie Steelsmith, ND, LAc, a Honolulu-based naturopathic physician and coauthor of *Great Sex, Naturally: Every Woman's Guide to Enhancing Her Sexuality Through the Secrets of Natural Medicine.* She encourages today's sensual women to explore the following three anatomical wonders, alone and/or with a partner, experimenting to discover new sources of joy.

Secret #1: **There's more to the clitoris than meets the eye.** In addition to the visible "nub" (the clitoral glans), its protective hood and the clitoral shaft directly under the glans, the clitoris includes two wing-shaped "legs" or crura (the singular form of the word is crus). These reach downward and to the sides, along the pubic arch, for about four inches.

The clitoris also includes two vestibular bulbs, typically about three to five inches long, extending from the clitoral shaft and continuing along the sides of the inner labia and vaginal opening. The crura and bulbs are made of erectile tissue—which means that stimulation of those areas causes the tissues to swell with blood, leading to very enjoyable sensations.

Pleasure maximizer: "With gentle pressure and massage to the vulva, including the labia and clitoris, these underlying structures will be stimulated. Some women choose to use vibrators or other devices to increase sensation," Dr. Steelsmith said.

Secret #2: **The perineum (the area between the vagina and anus) provides another potential surprise because its midpoint is especially sensitive to touch.** Called the perineal sponge, it too swells up when you're aroused and feels wonderful when gently massaged or stroked.

What's more, Dr. Steelsmith said, according to traditional Chinese medicine, the center of the perineum is the site of an important acupressure point called Hui Yin. Pressing on this point can enhance sexual energy.

Dr. Steelsmith's suggestion: "This area can be directly massaged during foreplay or intercourse. Some women report very pleasurable sensations when firm, rhythmic pressure is used."

Secret #3: **Many women are unaware of the role that the urethral sponge—or G-sponge, to use the term coined by Dr. Steelsmith's coauthor and husband, Alex Steelsmith—can play in sexual fulfillment.** Located directly behind the G-spot, the G-sponge consists of erectile tissue and specialized glands that produce a fluid that some women ejaculate from their bodies when sufficiently aroused. "The G-spot earned its reputation for triggering orgasmic ecstasy only because pressing on it during arousal means stimulating the G-sponge," Dr. Steelsmith said.

To find the G-sponge, use your index or middle finger to reach one to two inches inside your vagina...curl your finger upward to feel along the center of the front vaginal wall...then press directly on the swollen, spongy area. Ejaculation happens, typically after some minutes of consistent stimulation, when intense muscular contractions squeeze the built-up fluid in the sponge into the urethra. Dr. Steelsmith explained that the fluid, though it does emerge from the urethral opening, is not urine. Rather, it is a clear and watery fluid with a pleasant musky aroma.

Enjoyment enhancement: "It is easiest to stimulate this special area with a finger or a vibrator. And it is often stimulated by a man's penis during intercourse, especially if he is entering the woman's vagina from behind," Dr. Steelsmith said. It's well worth giving this a try—because when G-sponge stimulation leads to female ejaculation, the release may be accompanied by an orgasm that is deeply intense and immensely satisfying.

Have Much Better Sex As You Age

Dagmar O'Connor, PhD, sex therapist in private practice in New York City. She is the creator of a self-help sex therapy video or DVD and book packet *How to Make Love to the Same Person for the Rest of Your Life—and Still Love It. DagmarOconnor.com.*

Most older Americans grew up not talking about sex. Through others' silence, they were taught to believe that sex was shameful and taboo. Any mention of sex between "old folks," in particular, made people shudder.

Sexual activity is a natural and healthy part of life. In fact, you can get better at sex and enjoy it more—at any age. I treat couples in their 80s and 90s who wouldn't dare tell their children or grandchildren that they're seeing a sex therapist. Typically, whatever the state of their sex life, therapy improves it.

With retirement's gift of time, you can learn how the aging body works differently from its younger self, what pleases you individually and how to please each other in new ways.

PRACTICAL MATTERS

Yes, bodies change with age. Many women start to feel old and asexual at menopause. Men may develop erectile problems. But most difficulties can be overcome.

Physical change: Chronic conditions, such as diabetes, thyroid disease, cancer, Parkinson's disease and depression, can affect sexual function. With heart disease, sex can cause chest pain, and with asthma, breathlessness.

Remember, intercourse is the equivalent of walking two city blocks. Check with your doctor first.

Physical change: Joint pain and stiffness from arthritis makes sex difficult.

Solution: Relax in a Jacuzzi or bath before sex...vacation together in a warm climate... find new positions that won't stress your sore spots.

Physical change: Many drugs—antidepressant, hypertension, heart disease and some cancer medications, as well as alcohol—can affect sexual function.

Solution: If your sex drive is down or you're having other sexual problems, ask your doctor whether your medications could be the cause and if switching might help.

Physical change: After menopause, vaginal tissue becomes less elastic, the vaginal opening becomes smaller and lubrication decreases.

Result: Discomfort during intercourse.

Solution: Don't avoid sex—increase it. The more tissue is exercised, the more it stretches and the more you relax your muscles. Using your finger or a dildo, gently widen the vaginal opening every day. If the problem persists for more than two months, see a gynecologist or sex therapist.

Meanwhile, smooth the way with a nonprescription water-based lubricant, such as Astroglide or K-Y Jelly.

Not as good: Oil-based lubricants or petroleum products such as Vaseline. They may linger in the vagina and irritate it.

Bonus: Applying lubricant may get you in the mood for sex. Or let your partner apply it as part of lovemaking. Good foreplay makes lubrication flow naturally.

Physical change: With age, men require more manual stimulation for erections, take longer to ejaculate and have a longer refractory period—the amount of time between an orgasm and the next erection.

Solution: Patience. These changes are an invitation to discover the slow, loving sex that many women, in particular, have always wanted but haven't received.

Erectile problems can be treated medically, too. Discuss the situation with your doctor. You may be referred to a urologist for medication or other treatment.

BEYOND INTERCOURSE

Couples in their 60s and 70s and older often ask me what to do about erectile problems and other issues that interfere with intercourse. I tell them to slow down—expand their sexual horizons, develop new sexual habits and start all over again. The goal is simply to feel more.

Our society fears low-level arousal—pleasurable excitement that doesn't lead to penetration or orgasm. But those who have always resisted "just touching" become gluttons for such physical connection once they realize how great it is.

Exercise: During the day or with a light on at night, one partner lies back and is touched by the other—but not on the breasts or genitals—for 15 minutes to an hour. The person being touched stipulates what's wanted in a non-verbal way. If you would like your partner to touch more slowly, put your hand over your partner's and slow it down. When the "touchee" is finished, switch places.

Simple interludes set a loving, sensual tone and encourage you both to overcome shyness about requesting what pleases you. Prolonged sensual touching without genital contact removes sexual anxieties…helps you become relaxed, sensitized and responsive…revives a sense of trust and well-being that you may not have experienced since you were stroked as a child.

146

You'll emerge from the interlude feeling wonderful about each other. Resentments and recriminations will evaporate. Making sensual, uninhibited love often follows naturally. If not, there's always next time.

LOVE YOUR BODY AS IT IS

Our society presumes that only the young and skinny are (or should be) sexually active. As a result, many older people avoid sex out of embarrassment about spotted skin, a protruding stomach, wrinkles and flab. (Do remember that while you are ashamed of your wrinkles and protruding belly, your partner's eyesight has probably also diminished!) A mastectomy or other surgery can interfere with self-esteem, too, especially with a new partner.

Your body is miraculous. Learn to love it the way it really looks. One woman attending my sexual self-esteem workshop said, "I did not learn to love my body until I lost it." But your body at any age is a gift. Value it for itself…not as it compares with anyone else's or to how you looked when younger.

Exercise: Stand together before a full-length mirror. Say what you like about your own body out loud. Do this exercise alone first, before sharing it with your partner. Then try the exercise with your partner, taking turns. Listen, but don't respond.

To learn to appreciate your body, admire it often. Come away from this event loving five things about your body.

If you look better, you'll feel better. I recommend exercise—walking, swimming, Pilates—to couples of all ages. Getting stronger makes both women and men look better and feel more powerful…more sexual.

EDUCATE YOUR PARTNER

The young body works without thought. As you grow older, you can—and may need to—benefit from learning more about your body and your lover's. The key to intimacy is to express your needs—once you have learned what they are—and to insist on knowing the needs of your partner so that you can try to fulfill them.

Special note to women: If you rarely initiated sex but would like to, take baby steps. Try asking for different ways of being touched, or take his hand and show him how you like to be touched.

Exercise: Turn up the thermostat, and hang out nude together. Sleep nude in the same bed even if you haven't done so for years.

When It Hurts to Make Love

Barbara Bartlik, MD, is a sex therapist and assistant clinical professor of psychiatry at Weill Cornell Medical College in New York City. She is the author of numerous scientific publications and medical advisor for the book *Extraordinary Togetherness: A Woman's Guide to Love, Sex and Intimacy.*

When it comes to sex, sometimes the spirit is willing but the flesh says, "Ow!" If lovemaking has become painful, see your gynecologist. *Possible causes…*

• **Dryness.** Insufficient vaginal lubrication can be caused by dehydration…side effects of birth control pills or antidepressants…and decreased levels of the hormone estrogen after menopause.

What helps: Drink 64 ounces of water daily. Try an over-the-counter (OTC) lubricant, such as Replens, available at drugstores. Extend foreplay to give your body time to create lubrication.

Prescription topical estrogen also can help. It is less likely than oral estrogen to increase risk for cardiovascular problems and breast cancer. Options include a vaginal estrogen cream or an estrogen-containing ring inserted into the vagina.

Recent research: A low-dose vaginal estrogen suppository or ring (about 10 to 25 micrograms) is as effective as a higher-dose product for relieving dryness yet is less likely to cause side effects, such as headache and breast pain.

• **Endometriosis.** When tissue from the endometrium (uterine lining)—which should stay inside the uterus—instead attaches itself to organs outside the uterus, it causes pelvic pain and inflammation for women in their reproductive years.

Options: Take an OTC nonsteroidal anti-inflammatory drug (NSAID), such as *ibuprofen* (Advil) or *naproxen* (Aleve), starting the day before your period is due and continuing until bleeding stops. To halt disease progression, your doctor may prescribe oral contraceptives. In severe cases, surgery to remove endometrial tissue and adhesions can relieve pain while preserving fertility—though symptoms may recur. If pain is extreme and you are done having children, you may want to consider a hysterectomy.

• **Pelvic inflammatory disease (PID).** A bacterial infection of the reproductive organs, PID results from a sexually transmitted disease (such as chlamydia or gonorrhea) or other vaginal infection. Repeated douching and using an IUD (intrauterine device for birth control) can increase risk. PID symptoms include painful intercourse, vaginal discharge and abdominal or back pain.

Caution: PID can cause scarring that leads to infertility and chronic pain. Antibiotics cure the infection but cannot reverse damage.

Your partner: He must see his doctor, even if he has no symptoms of infection (such as pain or discharge from the penis)—without treatment, he could reinfect you.

• **Trichomoniasis.** This parasitic infection usually is transmitted sexually but in rare cases can occur if genitals come in contact with an object that harbors the parasite, such as a wet towel. It causes vaginal odor, yellow-green discharge, sores on vaginal walls, genital itching and pain during sex.

Cure: One large dose of an antibiotic, such as *metronidazole* (Flagyl), can work as well as a seven-day lower-dose course of treatment —but it increases risk for side effects, such as nausea and vomiting. Your partner also must be tested.

• **Uterine prolapse.** This occurs when weakened muscles and ligaments of the pelvic floor allow the uterus to drop into the vagina, creating pressure in the vagina or a lump at the vaginal opening. Contributing factors include pregnancy, childbirth, obesity, chronic constipation and decreased estrogen.

Self-help: Kegel exercises strengthen the pelvic floor. Contract vaginal muscles as if to stop the flow of urine...hold five seconds... relax...repeat. Aim for 30 repetitions daily.

Treatment: Your doctor may fit you with a pessary—a flexible plastic device worn in the vagina to reposition the uterus. Some pessaries can be worn during sex. If a bulge protrudes from the vagina, your doctor may recommend surgery to repair the pelvic floor...or a hysterectomy.

●**Vaginismus.** Involuntary spasms of the pubococcygeus (PC) muscles surrounding the vagina make intercourse extremely painful. Possible causes include pelvic or vaginal infection or injury...lingering pain (or fear of pain)...hormonal changes...or psychological issues.

Relief: Treat any underlying physical cause —with medication to cure an infection or with hormone therapy for low estrogen. Kegel exercises, physical therapy and biofeedback help relax the PC muscles.

In the privacy of your home: Your doctor may recommend vaginal dilators, phallic-shaped rods of various sizes. Starting with the smallest (tampon-size), you gently insert the dilator into your vagina, working up to larger dilators over time until you can comfortably accommodate penetration by your partner.

●**Vulvodynia.** This chronic condition is characterized by stinging or stabbing pain in the vagina or vulva. The cause may be related to genetics...infection...or injury to vulvar nerves, such as during childbirth, especially if you had an incision or tear at the vaginal opening. There is no known cure.

What helps: Medication options include an anticonvulsant or tricyclic antidepressant to block pain signals...and injections of the anesthetic lidocaine. Physical therapy and biofeedback help relax pelvic muscles.

Avoid: Hot tubs, tight underwear, scented toilet paper and perfumed soaps.

For more comfortable sex: Apply a topical anesthetic, such as lidocaine cream, 30 minutes before intercourse. This will diminish sensations of pain (and also, unfortunately, of pleasure). Use a vaginal lubricant...and apply cold compresses after lovemaking.

More from Dr. Bartlik...

When to Consult a Sex Therapist

See a trained sex therapist (a psychiatrist, psychologist or social worker) if medical treatment does not ease pain...your doctor finds no medical cause for your discomfort... or you suspect an emotional cause for painful lovemaking. A sex therapist can suggest sexual techniques and positions that minimize discomfort...allow you to examine fears or relationship problems in a supportive setting... and help you change behaviors that interfere with pleasure. *Referrals...*

●**American Association of Sexuality Educators, Counselors and Therapists,** 202-449-1099, *aasect.org.*

●**Society for Sex Therapy and Research,** 847-647-8832, *sstarnet.org.*

Would Snooping Enhance Your Relationship?

Lauren Zander, cofounder and chairman, The Handel Group, New York City. *HandelGroup.com*

The right to privacy is so integral to us here in America that it is written into our constitution...and yet our resident life coach, Lauren Zander, says that it may be destructive to intimacy in romantic relationships. Now there's a controversial position to take! We don't expect everyone to be in total agreement with what she has to say on this particular topic, but we do think that she has some really interesting points to make that are, at the very least, worth thinking about if you want to achieve a deeper closeness with your significant other.

The very idea that someone else—even a loved one—might be "snooping" (a.k.a. looking at your e-mails, examining your credit card bills and reading your text messages) makes many people uncomfortable. But Zander says it is, for the most part, a good thing! There are some caveats to this—we'll get to those in just a bit—but by and large, she believes that such "snooping," when it's done by mutual consent, can and will make your closest relationships stronger, happier and more resilient. You'll talk more and fight less.

WHAT ARE YOUR DARKEST SECRETS?

According to Zander, people in intimate relationships often have secrets on a number of levels, for example, what they really think about their sex life together…how they talk about the other to their friends…what they write in their journals about the relationship…how they spend money on private splurges…and more. And that's why, in many cases, their partners start to secretly poke into their affairs—they have the feeling that their partner isn't being entirely honest with them and are worried about it. "In many cases," Zander told me, "people hide information from each other in a sincere attempt to keep the peace—but what they are, in fact, doing is setting the stage for trouble."

Let's step back for a minute and ask ourselves: Why do we think we need privacy in our most intimate relationships? You know the answer—it's because we don't want to deal with the other person's reaction if the private things were to become known. And that's exactly why Zander believes that "snooping" is productive and relationship-enhancing.

Zander points out that the real reason that people object to a partner's snooping has nothing to do with "rights"—it is that there are some things that they want to hide simply because they don't want to give them up. These may be behaviors that aren't necessarily destructive or evil but that nevertheless may rock the boat. Examples include a woman who is hiding her designer-shoe habit…a man who regularly visits "adult sites" online…or engaging (men and women equally!) in Facebook flirtations. And then sometimes, of course, discoveries can be really disturbing, such as if you find out that your partner is actually having an affair.

LIVING IN TRUTH

Whether big or little, all secrets and lies create dysfunction in a relationship, and it is only through truth that the partners can start to meaningfully negotiate their differences. Allowing your partner to have access to the real truth about who you are and what you do forces the two of you to talk about your desires, hopes and dreams and, yes, your unmet needs as well. That's a good thing for a couple, because then you can start figuring out how to meet them. Once you are doing that, the possibility of living a happy life together is within your reach. And that's why Zander encourages couples to make a mutual decision that from now on there is no hiding, including e-mails, text messages, credit card bills or anything else. She sums it up as "committing to living in a way that it doesn't matter if your partner snoops, because you have nothing to hide."

For snooping to be the kind that Zander supports, it must be open snooping—in other words, all parties have to know it is going on. "When the CIA snoops, we call it 'gathering intelligence,'" she says, "and everyone knows that is what our spies are doing. Good personal snooping is also gathering intelligence, but it concerns people who are important in your life."

The Surprising Reason Couples Fight

Yukio Ishizuka, MD, psychiatrist in private practice in Rye, New York. He is author of the eBook *Breakthrough Intimacy: Sad to Happy Through Closeness.*

When we argue with our partners, we typically attribute the fight to a recent incident. A couple might fight over who forgot to pay the utility bills or why they got lost during a drive.

What couples do not realize is that the event that seems to trigger a marital fight usually is just an excuse to argue, not the true root cause. The actual cause of fights between partners in close relationships may be closeness itself.

My research with hundreds of married couples has shown that fights are most likely when relationships reach new levels of closeness and intimacy. This increased closeness makes the partners feel more dependent on each other and, therefore, more vulnerable and threatened.

Example: A couple argues seemingly because a mother-in-law is coming for yet another visit. They do not realize that the real reason they are fighting is that they just had a romantic weekend and felt particularly close to each other, an unfamiliar feeling that left at least one of them feeling more vulnerable.

The good news is that arguments brought on by increasing closeness offer an opportunity for the couple to get even closer.

GETTING PAST FIGHTS

Four key steps to getting closer…

1. Recognition. The first step is recognizing warning signals, catching yourself in a familiar emotional confrontation with the very person that you care for the most. Recognize negative emotions, such as anxiety, anger and depression, as warning signals that you are facing a challenge.

2. Perspective. Consider why you are facing this challenge, what your options are for solving it and what the consequences are for each of those options. Recognize that closeness is the top priority over all other considerations, such as being right or wrong…or winning or losing an argument.

3. Decision. Should you apologize? Agree to forget the whole thing? The best decision is to take whatever action is necessary to overcome the crisis.

4. Action. Implement your decision to the best of your ability. Think, feel and act in ways that increase closeness. Sometimes all it takes is to say, "Sorry, I didn't mean any of those nasty things I said. I love you." Or simply reach out affectionately as if nothing had happened.

How Being Too Supportive Can Harm Your Marriage

Being too supportive may harm a marriage. Giving too much support—usually as unwanted advice—is a bigger risk factor for marital unhappiness than not giving enough support.

Reason: Someone who does not get enough support from a spouse can get more from family and friends—but someone who is given too much support cannot escape it.

Erika Lawrence, PhD, leader of a study of 103 husbands and wives, published in *Journal of Family Psychology*.

Working Out Can Bring on the Big O

Debby Herbenick, PhD, MPH, director of the Center for Sexual Health Promotion, an associate professor in the department of applied health science at the School of Public Health and a health and sexual health educator at the Kinsey Institute, all at Indiana University in Bloomington. She also is the author of *Sex Made Easy: Your Awkward Questions Answered—For Better, Smarter, Amazing Sex* and lead author of a study on exercise-induced orgasm published in *Sexual and Relationship Therapy*.

Most of us have our orgasms in bed… or maybe on the living room floor in front of a fire if we're feeling frisky. But would you have guessed that the gym is a Big-O hot spot? Well, it's true—and surprisingly common! And it has nothing to do with the presence of bare-chested, muscle-bound male personal trainers. Rather, it's because certain types of exercise can trigger orgasms in some women, a new study has found.

The online survey recruited participants via websites related to women's issues, fitness and sexual topics as well as via e-mail. Respondents included 530 women ages 18 to 64, most of whom were married or in a relationship. Exercise-induced orgasms were reported by 124 women (23% of survey respondents)…another 246 (46%) said they experienced exercise-induced sexual pleasure but not orgasm. Do those percentages sound high? The study wasn't designed to measure prevalence specifically, and researchers estimated that prevalence in the general adult female population is closer to 5% to 15%—but perhaps the phenomenon is more common than people realize because those who experience it keep quiet out of embarrassment. Indeed, the majority of orgasmic exercisers in the survey reported feeling self-conscious… though they also reported feeling happy about the experience.

Climax-producing moves: Among women reporting exercise-induced orgasms within the previous 90 days, 51% said the climaxes occurred while they were doing abdominal exercises. Other common triggers included Pilates (32%)…lifting weights (27%)…yoga (20%)…biking/spinning (16%)…running (13%) …and walking/hiking (10%).

What's up down there? Orgasm often is associated with fantasizing, but the orgasmic exercisers reported that they weren't thinking about sex while they were working out. One possible explanation for the phenomenon is that certain exercises work the muscles and stimulate the nerves of the pelvic floor, which in turn can enhance a woman's arousal. (Some men also climax while working out, a topic the researchers are studying currently.)

Intrigued? If you want, experiment with various abdominal exercises, such as crunches and sit-ups, which the survey showed were most commonly associated with exercise-induced orgasm. Participants also mentioned equipment called a captain's chair, which consists of a rack with back support and padded armrests that allow the legs to hang free. To use it, stand with your back pressed against the backrest, forearms on the armrests and hands gripping the handles…support your weight on your forearms as you bend both legs and raise your knees to your chest, keeping your legs together…then lower your feet to the floor…repeat 10 to 15 times. At the least, you'll wind up with fab abs—and maybe you'll get a secret bonus as well.